REASON TO SMILE

11 KEYS TO YOUR BEST ORAL HEALTH EVER

HOW TO CONFIDENTLY CHOOSE THE *BEST*
DENTAL CARE FOR YOUR FAMILY

TYLER WILLIAMS, D.D.S.

outskirts
press

Get Even More—
Register Now for Your Bonus Content!

To maximize your value from this book, we have created an online companion to help you see and feel what the latest advances in dentistry can do for you. The old way of dinosaur dentistry has been put to rest. You have better options than ever to obtain the smile you've longed for.

Register your book at https://www.pinecrestdds.com/book-extras to unlock insider access to:

- How-to videos
- Special oral health reports
- Exclusive offers
- Patient testimonials and success stories
- Real before and after photos
- Procedure videos
- Step-by-step home protection systems
- Much more

Visit https://www.pinecrestdds.com/book-extras to register your book today!

If you have questions, comments, or feedback, please email us at reservation@pinecrestdds.com. We look forward to seeing your smile soon.

Contact Us:

Pinecrest Dental

463 W Murray Blvd
Murray, UT 84123

Office: (801) 618-1501
Fax: (801) 405-7709

Email: reservation@pinecrestdds.com
Web: pinecrestdds.com/book-extras

Table of Contents

Preface:
Why a Book on Dentistry?

Thank you for reading this book. Because of a whole host of factors—including diets that are getting higher and higher in sugar and acid, misperceptions about oral health, and cost—dental disease is on the rise, and it affects all aspects of our health, which makes it even more imperative that we deal with it preventatively, immediately, and thoroughly. My goal with this book is to raise awareness about the benefits of great oral health and to help readers understand how preventative care can improve quality of life. Think of this as a handbook for oral systemic health for you and your family. Together, we can reverse the silent and powerful effects of dental disease. Together, we can save millions of dollars in avoidable health care costs in our communities while feeling great about our smiles.

If you want to take charge of your health and find out what you can start doing today, this book is for you. If you want to learn the daily practices that can save you or your family trips to the dentist or physician, this book can change your life. Most of all, if you feel you could benefit from a brighter smile, a better ability to chew, or a more comfortable mouth, then you will find this book valuable in your daily life.

My name is Tyler Williams, and I am a licensed, practicing dentist in Murray, Utah. I have been in practice since 2010 and have been fascinated with teeth, science, and smiles for many years. I grew up in Sandy, Utah, a suburb of Salt Lake County near Little Cottonwood Canyon. If you haven't visited there, you should. The views, snow resorts, and biking, hiking, and cycling are fantastic. I didn't know what I had right in front of me until I moved to a few other parts of the world. I'm so glad

I returned to raise my family here. When I'm not doing what I love in practice, my wife, kids, and I spend time enjoying the great outdoors that surrounds us.

I wrote this book because I have a passion for bringing positive change to the health of my patients, friends, and community. I have wanted to publish a book for several years. Knowledge only becomes power when we act. Because of years of school and practical work experience, I had the knowledge—and I'd taken my impact to a certain level because of my everyday work with my patients. But I wanted to amplify this action. Now I'm broadcasting the things I have studied, tested, and proven to those who are also ready to act. The Centers for Disease Control and Prevention (CDC) reported that nearly 40 percent of adult Americans had not seen a dentist in the past year (as of 2015 data). In fact, some estimates have been higher during economic downturns. It is a concern that in today's day and age, up to half of our population does not see the dentist regularly. In a study published in 2014, the Health Policy Institute of the American Dental Association (ADA) explained the top three reasons adults forgo dental care. They are:

1. Lack of perceived need for care
2. Cost of care, including having no insurance
3. Lack of time to get to a dentist

In this book, I show you that those three factors do not have to be barriers to a healthier mouth—and therefore a healthier body. My goal is for every American to have at least one dental checkup per year. This is a huge undertaking and will require years of work, more awareness, and thousands of helping hands. But I am confident this is an answer to our health care crisis, that it will dramatically lower costs for everyone, and most importantly, that it will make our lives richer. Optimal dental care is not about insurance benefits, extra expenses, or painful treatment. There are powerful things you can do at home that take only a few minutes each day—and sometimes no extra time at all—and can impact your health and lifestyle exponentially.

I thank God for giving me the opportunity to learn, study, struggle, study, learn more, and be able to share with others. I am thankful that I am always growing, not only as a doctor of dentistry but as a patient living the human experience myself. I thank my wife, Megan, and our three children for supporting me and for giving me extra motivation to write this book. I look forward to hearing about your personal success stories in better oral health.

ONE

Are the Two Silent Epidemics Affecting You?

Tooth Decay: As Common as a Cold

There is a proverb that states: "If the eyes are a window to the soul, then the mouth is the doorway to the body." One of the diseases that can do the most damage to the whole body is also one of the most common and most preventable: tooth decay. In fact, tooth decay is the *second most common disease in the United States*, next to the common cold. According to the National Institute of Dental and Craniofacial Research, 92 percent of adults have had, or will have, dental caries (cavities) in their permanent, adult teeth. Cavities are holes in teeth caused by decay. More than one in four adults have untreated decay and/or have three or more missing or decaying permanent teeth—and that's just some of the health issues they're probably suffering. The mouth and body are tightly connected— quite obviously, as the mouth is physically a part of the body, but also in ways we do not always observe, such as health links. Together, we can reverse the effects of this all-to-common disease. If you catch the decay before the cavity hurts, treatment is much less invasive, requiring much less time and cost to restore good health.

Decay Is a Chronic, Silent Disease...
And It's Ruining Smiles Right Under Our Noses!

Approximately 26 percent of adults are living with untreated cavities. Because we aren't going to the dentist regularly, too many of us unknowingly have cavities decaying our smiles. Others don't consider decay a major health issue, so treating it gets pushed off, for reasons we can all relate to. It's scary to deal with medical issues because of the perceived pain and cost, and we may remember from our childhoods the less than pleasant smell or taste of the dental office (times and technology have dramatically changed, by the way). Or we find ourselves getting so busy in our day-to-day lives that dental care gets put on the back burner. Plus, going to the dentist is not that exciting, right? And who wants to spend all of their discretionary income on getting their mouth worked on when there are music lessons to buy, vacations to fund, and fancy restaurants to try? It is important to remember, however, that a cavity is considered a chronic infection that is best addressed with prompt treatment. These holes won't close on their own and only get worse with time. But they can be prevented. In my experience of treating thousands of cavities, I have an incredibly high success rate, well over 95 percent. Your future self will thank you for acting now.

The Basics of Cavity Formation and Treatment

A cavity develops when a tooth decays from the outside in. Millions of bacteria are contained in the plaque that sticks to our teeth. We need bacteria in our mouth—they're part of a functioning oral system. But There are good and bad bacteria, just like everything else. By knowing how the bad bacteria gets there and how to avoid it, you can also feed the good bacteria. Considering all the bad bacteria possible in the mouth, yes, the oral environment is the dirtiest part of our bodies, for sure. Various risk factors contribute to turning the bacteria more harmful as it colonizes and grows. These include diet (for example, eating a lot of sugar), habits (such as not brushing regularly), and genetics (sometimes the odds are against you right out of the gates, but I'll talk about how to deal with that later). Harmful bacteria produce acid that eats away at teeth and causes cavities.

After the harmful bacteria create a cavity, the decay will continue to grow, causing permanent damage to the tooth and, if untreated, eventually requiring root canal treatment or tooth removal. If your dentist catches your cavity in the early stage, it can be treated with fantastic, newer technology: a bonded filling. This treatment involves removing the infected areas of the tooth, isolating, preparing and cleaning the area, and then sealing the cavitation with a strong resin composite that is lifelike in its look and feel. The best part is you can eat right away, without pain. You can enjoy the foods you love and be confident in how your teeth look.

Tooth Decay Can Harm the Whole Body—at Great Cost

Tooth decay can also seriously threaten the health of your entire body. It may be hard to imagine, but a tiny cavity in a tooth can be life-threatening. Remember, a cavity is a type of chronic infection. From a sensitive place like your mouth, which is integral with other major systems in your body, that infection can spread to the brain or heart. This is called a periapical abscess, a condition that begins as tooth decay and worsens to the point of life-and-death infection. When speaking at various schools to children, I often share the story of a twelve-year-old boy in Maryland who died from a toothache. He did not live in the 1700s, as one might guess, but in the 2000s. If his caregivers had taken him to the dentist when they first noticed an issue, his life could have been saved. For under $100, he could have been treated and made healthy again. Instead, over $200,000 was spent in the hospital trying to save him, and worst of all, he passed away. His story is so tragic—and avoidable. With the right knowledge and help, his tooth pain could have been prevented or treated without any compromise to his quality of life, let alone loss of it.

His is not a unique case. A Pew Charitable Trust study found that nearly 1 million Americans visit the emergency room each year due to dental pain, and the costs associated are estimated to be nearly $900 million. The number of ER visits due to toothaches, a common word for tooth root infections, is rising. Estimates show between 16 and 40 percent more ER visits because of toothaches occurring over a matter of a couple years. In other words, the seriousness of this health issue is increasing rapidly. This is alarming, and we need to reverse it.

I've seen countless patients who have wasted time at an ER before they came to me, when they should have been referred to a dentist to begin with. Don't get me wrong—emergency rooms save lives and provide a great service, when needed. However, they should not be needed for most basic tooth issues. And few have the resources to treat tooth pain. I've helped many patients who spend hours and hundreds or even thousands of dollars at an ER only to receive pain medication and antibiotics and be referred to a dentist for full treatment. In a modern dental practice, we can handle all of that under one roof, for a much lower cost than most hospitals and in much less time.

———— ◆ ————

Squash the Bugs You Share!

Did you know the cavity- or gum-disease-causing bacteria in your mouth can be shared? That's right, even through kissing and sharing utensils, destructive "bugs" in saliva can "jump" to someone else. If one partner has lots of cavities and kisses the other partner, who doesn't, the oral health of both partners can worsen over time. If a parent kisses an infant or toddler near the mouth, they can share the bacteria and dramatically increase the risk of the child developing Early Childhood Decay, a condition that develops before age five.

Unfortunately, I see these conditions in my office all too often. I'm not asking you to stop showing affection to your loved ones (but yes, if Grandma has lots of root canals and missing teeth, she should be aiming her kiss for Junior's forehead, not near his mouth!). But by intervening early, we've had great success helping individuals and families reverse these negative trends. Without acknowledgment or evaluation of a concern or possible problem, families end up paying extra hard-earned cash that they should spend on family activities.

———— ◆ ————

Know the Truth About Your Tooth

To further understand the damage a cavity can do to your tooth, let's go over some tooth anatomy. Think of a tooth like an egg with a hard and thin outer shell (for the tooth, this is the enamel, what keeps smiles white, bright, and healthy); the egg white, which makes up most of the egg (in the tooth, the dentin); and the soft center yolk (the pulp of the tooth). Once something penetrates the hard, protective outer layer, the vulnerable, softer inner layers are susceptible to harm.

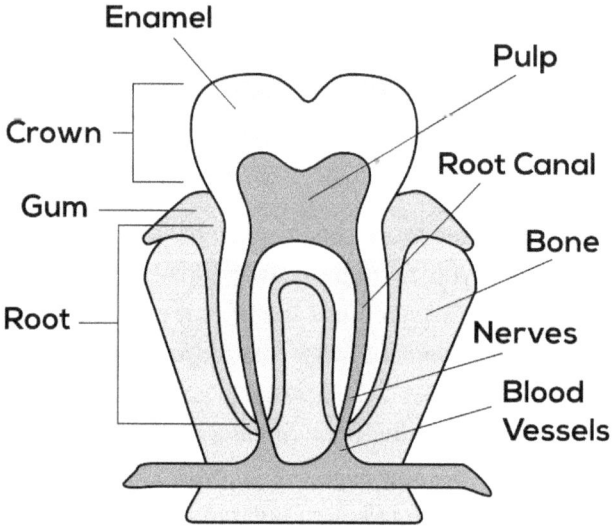

Tooth Anatomy

Never take your teeth for granted. They are wondrous parts of the body. Since teeth do not grow once they are fully erupted (grown in), they can last many years, if taken care of. They are also uniquely irreplaceable. Many other parts of our bodies can heal. Skin that is burned or cut can get better, sore throats go away, viruses attack and then leave, bones break and fuse back together...but teeth never grow back once they are lost. One day we may be able to mimic shark genes and grow more teeth in humans, but until then I'll impart some of my knowledge to help you or someone you care about to preserve that precious smile.

Many times I've had a patient in pain ask, "If I take antibiotics, won't my tooth get better?" The answer is always no.

Medications can mask some tooth problems for up to a few

weeks, even years, in rare situations. However, if a root cracks or a tooth is knocked out and not addressed quickly, it is lost forever. When a nerve dies or a tooth is damaged, it is a sitting duck for further infection. The blood supply is cut off from the vital inside of the tooth—so medications cannot physically reach the vital parts. No blood supply, no communication. Modern dentistry has taken a much more preventative and proactive approach than medical professionals of yesteryear. I am an "enamel worshipper" of sorts because I am incredibly appreciative what our Maker did to give us these teeth—in other words, naturally, all we need is right there—and it's our responsibility to take care of them. I want to help you understand how.

———— • ————

Let's look a little more at each of these layers, plus cementum, the tissue at the teeth's roots.

The hard and protective outer layer, called the enamel, is by far the hardest tissue in our bodies. Harder than our knees, our skulls, yes, even our elbows (which I know is hard to believe when your kid flings an arm your way in the middle of sleep). It is 96 percent inorganic, made up of hydroxyapatite, a crystalline structure of calcium and phosphorus. The rest of enamel is made up of organic material and water. This is why we don't "feel" decay until it gets bad—the hard outer layer of our teeth is like rock, which doesn't contain feeling or nerves and therefore has little ability to alert us of any changes taking place.

The enamel is the tooth's first line of defense against cavity-causing bacteria. If treatment is postponed, the bacteria will eventually get through the enamel and enter the layer of dentin and, eventually, the pulp. If cavity-causing bacteria gets that far, it can lead to a condition known as pulpitis, or inflammation of the pulp. This is the final warning before the pulp is irreversibly damaged. Early on, pulpitis can be treated with a bonded filling or restoration. If it's left to progress, more aggressive measures may need to be taken, such as a root canal or tooth extraction.

The middle layer, called dentin, is slightly harder than bone, but it is much softer than enamel. It is about 45 percent inorganic minerals, 30 percent organic matrix, and 25 percent water. Dentin is naturally yellow, so if the enamel wears away or is eroded, teeth appear yellower. The dentin makes up the bulk of our tooth by volume.

The inner layer is called the pulp, which contains the tooth's blood vessels and nerves. This is the pain center that lets us know when a tooth is worn, damaged, or affected by gum disease, or when decay is spreading. The "alarm" inside warns us to the most vulnerable areas of our teeth, so we know when and how to act.

Finally, there's a tissue called cementum, which covers the roots of the teeth and helps anchor the teeth into the jaw and attach them to the gums, so they function properly. When gums recede, or we become "long in the tooth," then, thousands of microscopic nerves covering our cementum are exposed, which may cause sensitivity, increased risk for decay, and a higher chance of tooth loss. Cementum is also naturally yellow, and its exposure is one of the biggest oral comfort and health challenges for longer-living adults.

More Resources than Ever, but Still Unhealthy

The midtwentieth century witnessed phenomenal improvements in technology and access to better oral health. In 1938, the nylon toothbrush arrived in stores; by 1961, the United States was enjoying cordless, rechargeable electric toothbrushes, developed in Switzerland after World War II. In 1945, Grand Rapids, Michigan, was the first city to add sodium fluoride to public water systems; by 1950, fluoride was an ingredient in many toothpastes. In 1948, President Harry S. Truman signed a Congressional bill establishing the National Institute of Dental Research and initiating federal funding for dental research.

It's hard to imagine, but one hundred years ago, only seven out of one hundred American households had toothpaste in their medicine cabinets. Can you imagine if only a select few of your friends brushed their teeth? Yuck! My wife wouldn't have gone on very many dates with me back then. Thanks to Claude Hopkins, an advertising executive for Pepsodent in the early 1900s, American households with toothpaste in their medicine cabinets leaped from 7 percent to 65 percent by the 1950s.

The most common reason for World War II draft rejection was the would-be soldier having too few teeth because he had problematic dental decay. The National Institute of Health (NIH) found that, back then, three out of ten Americans (17 million total) had lost all their teeth by age forty-five. With the requirement that military recruits brush and with toothpaste becoming more popular for the masses, things began to change. The jingle *"You wonder where the yellow went when you brush your teeth with Pepsodent"* and a minty taste added to toothpaste took brushing mainstream and changed the way we view home oral hygiene in the twentieth century.

Yet by 2011, most American adults—91 percent of those aged twenty to sixty-four—still had tooth decay (reported by the NIH and the CDC). Beyond age sixty-five, that number jumped to 95 percent.

So why are we seeing such high levels of decay today if fluoride and toothpaste are so readily available? Dental decay still affects over 90 percent of Americans, disproportionately in certain age groups and populations. Shouldn't we be healthier?

I believe our American diet is largely to blame. Soft drinks are easier than ever to access, often easier to find than clean, safe drinking water. Energy and diet drinks have grown in popularity and are full if acidic additives that wreak havoc on the oral cavity and overall health. I can't count the number of patients I've seen with "Mountain Dew mouth" from drinking sodas daily. Many people have no idea how bad they are for our teeth. Similar effects come from adding citrus such as lemons and limes to beverages. Sports drinks such as Gatorade and Powerade are just as bad, or worse.

In my late twenties, while in dental school, I tried a new and popular energy drink on an empty stomach, before a late road trip. It was a bad idea: don't try this at home. Within minutes, my heart was pounding and my stomach was in knots. That's when I decided I would avoid energy drinks completely. Today, I only consume soda occasionally on week-ends. I call it being a "social drinker" of carbonated drinks. I've seen too many patients destroy their smiles, slowly, silently, and often irreparably. When we are able to correct the damage, it takes incredible time and money, expenses that can be avoided through lowered consumption of sugar and acid, which often comes in the form of beverages.

Don't Just Treat Decay—Prevent It

One of the ways we can improve our health and lower our health care spending is through prevention. Today, we have excellent newer and safer technology to aid in cavity prevention.

Let's "Seal the Deal" on Better Health

Sealants are one such preventative service. The chewing surfaces of our teeth are covered in deep and narrow grooves and crevices that trap cavity-causing bacteria. For a metaphor, think of steep mountains and narrow valleys—when a large rock rolls down into a valley, it does not easily roll out, because of the steep mountains. Our teeth's natural grooves are often too narrow for food particles to escape, too narrow even for a toothbrush to clean well. When we seal teeth, we clean or lightly prepare the stained grooves, and then we bond a resin sealant coating in the grooves to make the tooth glassy-smooth.

Many people receive sealants between age six and twelve, as adult teeth begin to grow in, but we seal adult teeth now as well. People love it because it's the new way to avoid a cavity altogether (as long as you keep up with the maintenance of continuing to brush your teeth and visit the dentist). A study in Australia found a single sealant can provide up to fifteen years of benefits. There are no car tires available today that last that long and for such a relatively inexpensive price. Even if it wears out after ten or fifteen years, a sealant has done its job incredibly well as it has saved you from a root canal or broken tooth. The cost of sealants are pennies on the dollar compared to what a root canal may cost. We are now sealing older resin fillings and even certain front teeth with deep grooves as well. My molar teeth were sealed when I was in early elementary school, and I have had several resealed in recent years. My healthiest patients usually choose to do the same. It's painless, and it takes under twenty minutes to seal one tooth. This is preventative dentistry at its finest!

Varnish: The Two-Minute Mineral Application That Could Save Your Smile

The latest preventative measure is to give your teeth a direct coating of minerals through a fluoride varnish. The application contains a high amount of fluoride minerals, over 22,000 parts per million, compared to over-the-counter toothpaste, which is at 1,000 parts per million. (Tap water is just under 1 part per million, which I discuss elsewhere in this book.) Varnish may also contain calcium and/or xylitol, depending on the brand. It is effective, safe, and easy to use. It is painted directly on your teeth, and you avoid eating for thirty minutes and brushing for four to six hours after the application. The topical use means it is applied right where it needs to go, without you swallowing it. It is great for both adults and kids, especially those who have a high risk of tooth decay.

When I was a kid, a fluoride treatment after my dental cleaning meant foam trays of goo placed in my mouth and a suction straw that I had to hold in place. I had to bite down for less than five minutes, but it felt like an eternity! Plus, while the fluoride was supposed to taste like bubble gum or berry, it really tasted like bad cough syrup. Today, varnish is tooth colored and makes your teeth feel a bit "fuzzy" for a few hours, but it brushes right off the next morning and you don't have to wait for it to start working.

The results I've experienced in my own practice were confirmed in a University of Florida study back in 2000. Some of our adults at highest risk for decay have it placed on their teeth every few months; others receive it with their semiannual dental evaluation and preventative cleaning. The coating helps reduce and prevent decay, dramatically decrease root sensitivity, and remineralize damaged surface enamel. The best part? Studies show the benefits last from three to six months with just one application. That's real dental insurance! It's so great, I have it applied to my own teeth at least three times per year for added protection, and it's helped my kids keep the "bad bugs" away too.

Don't Ignore—Treatment Is Better Than Ever

Sometimes you can't prevent damage from tooth decay, but the good news is that treatment options these days are astoundingly painless, effective, and accessible.

No More Fillings: How to Fix the Gap in Health Care

Once a tooth is sensitive or uncomfortable, you have moved well be-yond the preventative stage. Next time you need a cavity restored, ask your provider if resin bonding, the new alternative to silver fillings, is right for you. Amalgam silver has been around for many years; it's a long-lasting material and has saved many teeth over the past decades. When I've been out on mission service projects in rural parts of the United States and overseas, I've seen the benefit of this relatively in-expensive product, which can be placed quickly and without as much technique as bonded resins require. But newer ways are even better. Amalgam fillings are a combination of silver, tin, copper, zinc, and a small amount of mercury (the mercury allows the material to remain in a liquid form while it is applied to the tooth). Amalgam is now banned in parts of Europe due to worries over mercury ending up in the water systems. In the United States, we now have suction filters or amal-gam separators in our vacuum lines in dental offices to ensure proper disposal. Still, I now provide only resin restorations to patients in my office for a few reasons. These are:

1. The preparation of the tooth required for silver fillings is more invasive and aggressive. We can now add years to a tooth by taking out only the bad parts and bonding to the good ones. Modern dentistry is about saving as many teeth as possible, and bonding fits very well into this model.

2. Resin restorations chemically bond to teeth, which protects from sensitivity and adds strength.

3. There is no more "galvanic shock" or sensitivity from the ex-pansion and contraction of the metal with certain foods or eating utensils.

4. Resin restorations are gentler on your teeth than the fillings of old. My patients are consistently amazed at how smooth and comfortable the service is, all in one simple visit! Plus, there's

usually little or no sensitivity afterward, and you can eat right away.

5. People generally prefer the tooth-colored resin as an added benefit. You can choose to have it match the natural color of your teeth, or you can choose to have it whiter.

In my practice, resin bonding is the number one way we've been able to save more teeth from cracking and painful root canals. They look better than silver fillings, and they resolve the issue of annoying food traps. When under 50 percent of the total tooth volume needs restorative help, it's usually the best option. Bonding is only getting better as technology develops and resins become stronger and more lifelike. Plus, it's exponentially cost-saving to have bonding done before the tooth gets to the point of hurting. My patients are consistently amazed at how smooth and comfortable the service is, all in one simple visit!

Crowns Are Dead!

When a tooth is cracked, decayed, or severely damaged, it requires restorative treatment to treat it and avoid further damage. However, often a crown isn't the best option, especially on a virgin tooth. I place only one or two new crowns a month in my practice, usually only to replace old, worn-out crowns on teeth that are decayed underneath. Way too often I see crowns done in situations the patient could have chosen a more conservative option. It can be too hard for a patient to completely clean and maintain a tooth with a crown on it. With conservative ceramics and tooth-saving techniques, I have personally saved hundreds and hundreds of teeth using this technique

Twenty years ago, the technology for a ceramic onlay wasn't even close to where it is today, so your dentist really helped you by placing a conventional crown—it was the best technology at the time. I've seen patients with gold crowns that are over forty years old that are still functioning with great integrity. But we have advanced far beyond the excessive reduction of a tooth to a stump, which removes 60 to 70 percent of the natural tooth structure, leaving no enamel and very little dentin behind. Today, even when a conventional crown procedure is performed, we are much more conservative, thanks to modern methods and preparation.

If you have new damage to a tooth that doesn't already have a crown, consider a procelain onlay as great option. It could add decades to the life of your tooth. Depending on the extent of the damage, you have a few choices. We have found that when 50 percent or less of the tooth is decayed or cracked, a bonded resin filling, done in just one simple visit, is a great option. However, when the damage crosses the 50 percent volume threshold, a one-piece construction porcelain or ceramic restoration may be your best option. Even gold might work—that's right, gold is still a great material in certain situations. Our enamel never grows back, so saving as much of it as possible will preserve more of your tooth, leave it with more natural strength, and dramatically reduce the chance of the tooth needing a root canal. Plus, if the tooth requires more care years down the road, you could always place a larger onlay or a full crown on the tooth. Think of an onlay as a roof, compared to a crown as a roof with four walls. If you have to remove or replace the walls in your home, that could weaken the support for the roof. Plus, once we remove the "walls" that nature gave you, (whether by tooth decay, cracking or crown preparation) we can never make them as strong as they once were. With today's technology, less is more!

If a small leak happens in your home's roof, you can usually repair the shingles or a portion of the structure without replacing the whole roof. But if most of the roof is damaged, you may be better off not with lots of little patches but with a new roof. But just because you need a new roof, that doesn't mean you need to replace the exterior walls as well, right? That's where a full crown may be overkill – too much of your natural tooth removed, that could have been restored with a ceramic onlay instead. Plus an onlay is stronger and easier for you to maintain and clean.

An onlay is usually better than a crown in these situations for five reasons:

1. An onlay saves more of your enamel compared to a conventional crown.

2. Onlays are bonded to your teeth, creating a moisture-tight seal and added strength.

3. Onlays have margins (the area where the restoration meets your tooth) in more cleanable areas, above your gums, compared to a traditional crown.

4. Onlays match your natural tooth very well, or you can choose to have them made whiter.

5. Onlays are monolithic, which means they are strong because they are one material the whole way through.

Modern ceramics have come a long way. Years ago, they had to be laminated to look like real teeth—which means that the porcelain tooth covering alone wasn't strong enough, so it had to be veneered over the top of a gold or metal substructure. If you have an old crown, it may look gray or dark at the gumline. That's the metal showing through after years of wear. Modern resins have come a long way too. Fusing these two technologies (resins and ceramics) allows us to bond the new restoration to your natural tooth, which should provide years of lasting protection as long as you do your part to maintain it well at home and see your dentist for regularly scheduled maintenance. No more gray gumlines or dark teeth and a more natural and smoother finish.

Gum Disease: The Silent Thief of a Healthy Mouth

Periodontal disease, more commonly referred to as gum disease, is a condition caused by the breakdown of the tissues around your teeth. Over time, the increasing loss of bone and gums usually results in the total loss of teeth. Most of us think of cavities as the main cause of tooth loss. However, periodontal disease is the leading cause of tooth loss in adults, even more so than dental decay.

Nearly 50 percent of American adults have periodontal disease, which accounts for close to 65 million people. The number of affected people increases to over 70 percent for those sixty-five and older. Countless medical studies have also linked it with total-body issues, such as stroke, heart disease, cancers, erectile dysfunction, diabetes, Alzheimer's, arthritis, and infertility. Harvard ran a study a few years ago and found people with periodontal disease are at an alarming 63 percent greater risk to develop pancreatic cancer, one of the most aggressive and rapid cancers taking lives today.

Bleeding Equals Vulnerability

Bleeding gums are not OK! If your hands bled every time you washed them, you would be concerned. Not only does this mean your gums are not healthy but your blood vessels are left open and vulnerable to attacks from your oral environment. The implications go way beyond the mouth, circulating around all major systems of the body. A study by the Royal College of Surgeons in the United Kingdom showed that *Streptococcus gordonii*, the bacteria found in dental plaque, can produce a surface molecule that mimics a blood-clotting factor in the body called fibrinogen. This study found that *S. gordonii* would further cause blood platelets to aggregate, leading to a life-threatening blood clot. When our gums are healthy, and not bleeding, the bacteria cannot access the portal into our blood vessels.

Causes of Periodontal Disease

To prevent gum disease, it is important to assess the risks that can lead to its causes.

- Gum disease can be caused by restricted saliva flow. Countless prescription and over-the-counter medications cause dry mouth symptoms. Dry mouth (or xerostomia, as we refer to it clinically) decreases the amount of important minerals in the mouth, therefore weakening teeth and creating an acidic environment where decay-and-disease-causing bacteria thrive. Dry mouth irritates our gums, exposes our porous tooth roots, and increases bleeding.
- Hormonal changes in females could increase their risk for gingivitis, a precursor to periodontal disease. Examples of specific hormonal changes affecting women are pregnancy and menopause.
- Gum disease can be caused by genetic predispositions. Some individuals tend to be more genetically inclined to gum disease than others. If your parents, siblings, or grandparents had missing teeth or wore dentures, you are likely at an increased risk to lose teeth or develop periodontitis.
- Treatments for head and neck cancers can lessen saliva flow and the ability to eat and swallow, potentially leading to gum disease.
- People who suffer from diabetes are at a higher risk for infections, which includes gum disease. These two conditions have a very high correlation, and I see them coupled in my own practice daily.
- People with heart disease or high blood pressure have an increased risk for gum disease and for worsening heart conditions when gum disease is untreated.
- Smoking is a major risk factor for gum disease. Besides the vast array of other illnesses that could potentially arise from smoking, it can directly cause gum disease and lower the chances for

a successful treatment of the disease. Chewing tobacco also increases your risk for gum disease and oral cancer.

General Treatment

Today, our first line of care is nonsurgical. Most of my patients are amazed at how comfortable the treatment is. Mild local anesthesia is typically used, unless you are nervous and would prefer to be sedated. Most people can eat and drink comfortably the same day. For those with advancing periodontal conditions, we have home gel tray therapy and special mouth rinses to take extra precaution without surgery. We call this initial periodontal therapy.

For progressive or advanced periodontal disease, we have been successfully using a pain-free home tray system called Perio Protect. When you have periodontal disease, the bacteria that live in your gums and jawbone are classified as anaerobic, which means "without oxygen." This means that when these bacteria are exposed to oxygen for a constant period of time, they will break apart and die, so your gums can get healthy again. With Perio Protect, we make special lab-fabricated clear dental trays that our patients wear fifteen to thirty minutes per day. The trays are nearly invisible, so you can wear them while in the shower or while running errands. The special tray-gel combo creates a light hydraulic pressure that pushes a prescribed peroxide gel underneath your gums, which destroys the nasty bacteria causing your gum disease by forcing oxygen into them. Painlessly and comfortably you can help accelerate the gum therapy you receive at the dental office. The only side effect we've found with a system like this is whiter teeth, from the peroxide—and most people don't object to that! In the future, technologies such as oral probiotics and nanotechnology may be valuable tools to help us in periodontal therapy.

The Four Stages of Disease and Treatment

Now that I've spoken about gum disease in general, let's talk about its four distinct stages:

Gingivitis: This is the first stage of gum disease. It is the inflammation of the gums that is caused by the buildup of plaque and/or poor oral hygiene along the gumline, where each of your teeth meet your gums. We see it a lot in teens (especially those who wear braces and don't brush) and in young to middle-age adults. This stage usually develops when you have poor brushing and flossing techniques and when you skip your dental cleaning appointments. Gingivitis can usually be reversed with improvements in your oral hygiene routine and by receiving a professional cleaning or scaling. Tens of millions of Americans suffer from gingivitis. This is the "red in the sink" stage where you may have bleeding when you eat, floss, or brush. Bleeding happens in other stages as well, but if you are bleeding now, take action and you can reverse this, and you may avoid the next stages, which are irreversible.

Early Periodontitis: This is the second stage of gum disease. It involves the bacteria in the mouth spreading into the gums and underlying bone. When this happens, the gums, ligaments, and jawbone become so irritated that they start to separate and move away from the teeth. This forms pockets that tend to trap plaque and food particles, causing infection. This is the first irreversible stage of gum disease, but if taken care of early, we can arrest your disease together and have a healthy and comfortable outcome.

Progressive Periodontitis: This is the third stage of gum disease. It involves further invasion of the pockets between the teeth and gums and bone. The ligaments are further broken down, and the bacteria grows more rapidly. Usually breath worsens, as the higher levels of bacteria reproduce in the pockets around gums, and sensitivity increases, but not always. Our in-office evaluations find more bleeding in this stage and loose or mobile teeth.

Advanced Periodontitis: This is the fourth and most severe stage of periodontal disease. It involves the bacteria in your mouth further destroying the bone and ligaments that hold your teeth in place. We also find white blood or "pus" when we measure the pockets surrounding your teeth. If not treated quickly, tooth loss is inevitable. This is frustrating for both patients and doctors, because my goal is to save your tooth whenever reasonably possible. This often results in shifting, loose, and/or lost teeth. At this point, we must consider either surgery to save or implants to replace teeth. Malnutrition may become a problem as eating whole foods becomes more difficult. This can severely affect the ability to chew and smile, as well as overall health.

Again, today, our first line of care for most periodontal cases is nonsurgical. For those with advanced periodontal conditions, we utilize added home therapy and special mouth rinses to take extra action without surgery. For certain cases, however, we work with a periodontist to get our patients the best care. Periodontists can provide gum grafting, a procedure where receded or thin gums can be augmented to restore comfort and periodontal attachment to the teeth. Think of it like plastic surgery for your gums. This is a great service and can really help cover up those yellow, rough, and exposed roots that are prone to decay and erosion.

Speaking the Language of Periodontics

I asked my friend and colleague, Dr. Dan Thunell, to write on his experience working with gum disease in his periodontal practice. Dan is not only a great person but a skilled clinician. In fact, Dan has done several gum grafts on me. In my early twenties, I began to notice recession (I have a family history of gum recession), and I thought I should scrub harder to keep my teeth cleaner. Boy, was I wrong! (This was before I was in dental school and knew better.) As I mentioned, I believe this is one of the most helpful services a good periodontist can offer. When I have a patient with complex gum needs, especially when gum appearance or severely exposed roots come into play, Dan and I work together to help our patients get a great outcome. Here is a bit more about Dan.

An Exciting Time to Be a Part of Dentistry: Dan Thunell's Story

My name is Dan Thunell. I grew up in several different cities along the East Coast, but I call Atlanta, Georgia, my hometown. I attended Brigham Young University (BYU), where I attained a BA in linguistics, studying Italian and Arabic. There was no single tract to dental school at BYU, so I could study whatever interested me while simultaneously completing my requirements for entrance to dental school. I next attended the University of Pittsburgh School of Dentistry, where I received my DMD degree, and I then completed a Certificate in Periodontics at the University of Iowa. I am a husband, the father of six kids, and an avid cyclist, and I love my job.

I can't remember ever not wanting to be a dentist. My grandfather was a dental lab technician, and I remember playing with his tools in his basement as a young boy. My dad had some really crooked teeth, and I wanted to become a dentist or an orthodontist, so I could straighten them.

Once in dental school, I began my rotations through the various clinics and was exposed to all the different fields within dentistry. I still remember my first experience performing a periodontal procedure and thought it was the next best thing to sliced bread. While I may have entered dental school wanting to be an orthodontist, I left certain that periodontics was where I belonged. I enjoy the science behind periodontics and the oral-systemic link between periodontal conditions and other systemic health conditions. It's challenging to put the pieces together, but it motivates me daily in my practice. Periodontics is a field that is constantly evolving, and it stimulates me to be a constant learner and researcher. I believe the day is not too far in the future that we will be able to grow new teeth when a bad tooth is lost. This is an exciting time to be a part of dentistry.

The Exciting World of Grafting

One of the amazing procedures we perform as periodontists is soft tissue grafting. This is where tissue is built up around a tooth to correct receding gums. While I enjoy most aspects of periodontics, this area is most exciting to me. Receding gums are common, and their cause is multifactorial. In other words, it is hard to put your finger on a single cause. A few of the many causes include:

Tooth position in relation to the jaw bone: If the tooth is sitting at the extremes of or even outside the jawbone, this puts stress on the gum tissue around the tooth. Over time, this stress often results in the gumline receding or dropping, exposing the root of the tooth. Many people are born with "thin" gums. It's genetic and not something we have much control over. Thin gums are more prone to recession especially if tooth movement puts stress on them.

Aggressive brushing: We live in a busy society, and there never seems to be enough time to do everything on our checklist. Regular and correct brushing of our teeth is one of those checklist items that is often glossed over. We hurriedly scrub our teeth and press hard enough and go fast enough (we think) to get done in thirty seconds what should normally take two minutes. We are almost all guilty of this at times, and our gums can suffer as a result. This habit can damage the gums around the teeth, causing them to recede. It also prevents the active ingredients of toothpaste from reaching important spots on the teeth.

Clenching/Grinding teeth: Along with our busy schedules comes stress, and one way many of us manage that stress is by clenching or grinding our teeth. For many of us, it is a subconscious habit; we aren't even aware we are doing it. But this habit can be very destructive to the tooth as well as cause recession of the gums. If you feel your teeth with your tongue along the space where the tooth meets the gums, do you feel a sharp ledge on the tooth? Does it feel like there is an indentation in the tooth itself? If so, you may be clenching or grinding. There are many ways to treat this, and if you do so, you'll be doing your gums a favor too.

Frenulum pull: A frenulum is a fold of tissue that helps attach structures together. In our mouths, we have several frenulums. Most notably are the frenulums between top and bottom front teeth. This fold of tissue extends up from inside the lip and comes to a point above or sometimes at the level of the gumline. Other smaller frenulums exist in the mouth, as well as a large one under the tongue that secures the base of the tongue to the floor of the mouth.

The root of the tooth is much softer than the enamel, which makes up the top (or crown) of the tooth. To prevent decay, or further loss of the supporting structures of the tooth, a tissue, or gum graft is placed to build up the lost gum tissue and cover the exposed root. What many people don't realize is that as the gum recedes away from the tooth, the bone around that tooth is also receding under the gum tissue. This causes the tooth to become weaker and more susceptible to other problems down the road. Individuals with dry mouths are particularly susceptible to cavities on the roots of their teeth. Along with a proper oral hygiene program, a gum graft can be a real benefit for these individuals. If you have receding gums, let a dental professional evaluate them and see if a gum graft would be beneficial for you.

TWO

Five Steps to
Your Brightest Smile

Best-practice dental care is a lot like going to the gym. Every January, you renew your membership, not only for your long-term health but also to increase how you feel about yourself and your appearance. Not only do you feel better but you make better decisions and eliminate wastes and excess carbs and fats from your body. You can learn from trainers or other athletes on how to improve your technique, diet, and exercise routine.

A healthy mouth is critical for your overall physical wellness too. Many studies have linked disease and decay in the mouth to risk of disease elsewhere in the body. And just like you want a body that fits into your favorite pair of jeans, you want a smile that says who you are. After all, it's one of the first things people notice about you. A healthy smile boosts confidence and helps you feel proud when you say that first hello. In fact, *USA Today* ran a poll and found that a smile was the first thing most people notice when they meet someone. Even more noticed than hair, clothes, and eyes!

———— ◆ ————

There's No Time to Waste

Dental decay is the most common chronic disease in young people between the ages of five and seventeen, according to research by the CDC. Good oral health habits should be established early, so as children become teenagers, they have already established an effective oral hygiene routine and have a sound understanding of why it is important.

————◆————

Fortunately, while keeping a great smile does take daily maintenance, a preventative daily routine doesn't need to take long. Keeping up with it is the key, just as it is with diet and exercise. It's not just about getting in shape—it's about staying in shape! Here's my own routine I've tested and developed to strengthen my enamel, protect my gums, and make my smile naturally brighter. Create your healthy and happy smile with these five simple steps:

1. Start your day off bright: rinse with an anticavity (fluoride and xylitol) mineral mouth rinse when you first wake up. I also like to use a tongue scraper during this time.

2. Floss once daily. (More often is OK, but that's all you have to do—just once per day.)

3. Brush for two minutes after breakfast and before bed, preferably with a professional electric toothbrush for maximum results. Use soft bristles and massage at the gumline—don't scrub your teeth. Avoid eating, drinking, or rinsing for twenty minutes after brushing to maximize the mineral uptake on your teeth.

4. Drink water between meals.

5. Use xylitol products, such as mints, gum, or candies, throughout the day.

These five measures are safe yet powerful at keeping our mouths in tip-top shape. They also make weak teeth stronger. Don't worry—if you get off track in your daily home care, simply reup your commitment to these steps, and you can effectively reverse surface damage on your teeth before it comes irreversible decay. It can also help you reverse gingivitis before it becomes stage two, early periodontal disease. There was a period in my early adulthood when I had seven or eight new cavities in a row. Since then, I've developed this routine, and at the time of this writing, I've had seven years without a single new cavity.

Rinse

News flash: commercials are misleading! Rinsing with mouthwash should be the first thing you do at the sink, not the last. Most people use mouthwash after they floss and brush, just like on TV. It seems like a final breath freshener after a job well done. And it just feels good! But rinsing can move all the hardworking minerals in your toothpaste out of your mouth and into your sink before those minerals have finished penetrating and protecting your smile.

For a week, challenge yourself to rinse before you brush. Then see if you can do it for one week more…There are exceptions to this order of rinse first, floss and brush later, but for most adults and kids working on prevention, this is the best practice. Leave a film of paste behind to get a scaled-down version of after-the-dentist cleanliness at home. The coating is safe and effective because it's applied topically and directly to the area where it's needed most.

Floss

Flossing: the elephant in the room. Every time you open your medicine cabinet, there's a little plastic box of tightly coiled thread that we try to ignore, or we say, "I'll do it tomorrow." Most people don't floss regularly, unless there's a piece of food trapped. The problem is, tomorrow usually doesn't come. But flossing is one of the least expensive ways to prevent some of the most expensive dental care, and it only adds sixty seconds to your daily routine.

Your toothbrush can't reach everywhere in your mouth, like under the gumline and between your teeth. Brushing alone cleans only 60 to 70 percent of the surface area of your teeth. That means one-third or more of our precious enamel and root surfaces are missed when we skip flossing or don't do it correctly. Flossing removes bits of food and soft buildup and makes for a more complete cleaning of your teeth. I rate brushing alone, twice a day, without flossing, with a B- letter grade. Add in flossing, and that grade shoots up to an A. For my high-risk and most careful patients, we also add a Waterpik or AirFloss into their daily routine, rising their score to an A+ in defense.

Wait, the Government Said I Didn't Have to Floss...

In late 2016, flossing made news when the US government dropped its recommendation that people floss, citing a lack of evidence that the activity did any good. You may have thrown your floss in the trash or strutted into a dancing celebration when you read of the news!

Shortly after the story was released, my younger brother texted me and said, "Hey, did you read this?" with a link to the story. With a subtle grin, I invited him to stop flossing and see how his next dental checkup went. His response was "No way!" (He's a faithful flosser, by the way, and it's paid off well for him.) Countless studies, reports, and my own observation in my practice have demonstrated the benefits of flossing.

So, what's behind the idea that flossing does no measurable good? Some real-world studies are flawed because: (1) The funding isn't there to produce top-notch studies. And (2) comparing the effects of those who are flossing with those not flossing means we'd have to ask a group of people not to floss. Ethically, that's a problem. Asking people not to floss puts those people at great risk because flossing does prevent disease and decay, in my years of experience.

Six Steps to Flossing Right

The American Dental Association (ADA) continues recommending this low-cost and low-risk strategy. So do I. It's only harmful if you become overzealous in your flossing—and you won't do that if you follow this technique:

1. Once a day is all you need to be effective. This may take you less than ninety seconds. Can you spare that much time, as boring as it may be? If you have food traps or suffer with dry mouth, flossing two or three times per day may be helpful.

2. Pull out a long strand of floss (usually about eighteen inches). If you're flossing regularly, one of those travel packs your dentist gives you should last about a week.

3. Wind most of the floss around each middle finger, leaving an inch or two between your two fingers to floss with.

4. Now, get your thumbs and index fingers involved to maneuver the floss. Slide it down between two teeth, using a back-and-forth motion. Gently guide it around each tooth's base, under the gums. You may see or taste some blood. That's normal if you haven't flossed in a while, and you should see less and less red in the sink as you get into the flossing habit. After about a week of regular flossing, you won't bleed at all (unless you have periodontal disease).

5. Make a C-shape around each tooth as you glide up and down the gumline in a sweeping motion. You want to hug the neck of the tooth around the gums for best practice.

6. Use clean sections of floss as you move around your mouth.

———— ♦ ————

Floss Alternatives

If you think floss is boring or too difficult, you can still reap its benefits by using technology that mimics flossing. By themselves, these aren't quite as effective as flossing, but they still give oral health a huge boost and are much better than brushing alone. For maximum results, use an irrigator in the morning before brushing and then string floss before your nighttime brushing.

- *Oral Irrigator: Flossing the old-fashioned way can seem tedious. Using a water flosser is quicker and more fun. Even teenagers seem to love the idea of power washing their teeth.*

- *Shower Flosser: A spin on oral irrigation, the shower floss-er makes it even more convenient to floss your teeth. Simply attach an oral irrigation unit to your shower head for mess-free flossing. (Even if you don't want to install a shower attachment, you could still move your flossing routine to the shower. While your conditioner sets in, floss your teeth—my wife is a hair stylist, so I had to make a plug for hair care too...)*

- *AirFloss: Another alternative to conventional flossing, the AirFloss cleans out debris and plaque by shooting quick bursts of air and water in between teeth. You can add mouth rinse for a fresher cleaning. (I used this technique when I had orthodontics a few years ago, and it really helped keep my lunch out of my braces!)*

- *Waterpik: These devices look in some ways like an electric toothbrush but with a tube instead of bristles and hooked up to a water source. A forceful stream of water knocks the debris out from between your teeth.*

Irrigation really helped a family of six in my practice. They were pretty good about brushing, but flossing…not so much. One Christmas, the loving mom bought everyone Waterpiks. You know what happened? Well, first of all, they became obsessed with irrigating. The boys said they couldn't live without it anymore. And it resolved the gingivitis and bleeding between their teeth. Now, they weren't string flossing (yet!), so there was still some room for improvement, but hey, it was a huge leap toward better health. Best of all, they had a lot fewer cavities at each checkup, they felt better, and they had nice pink gums to show for it.

My Personal Flossing Moment of Truth

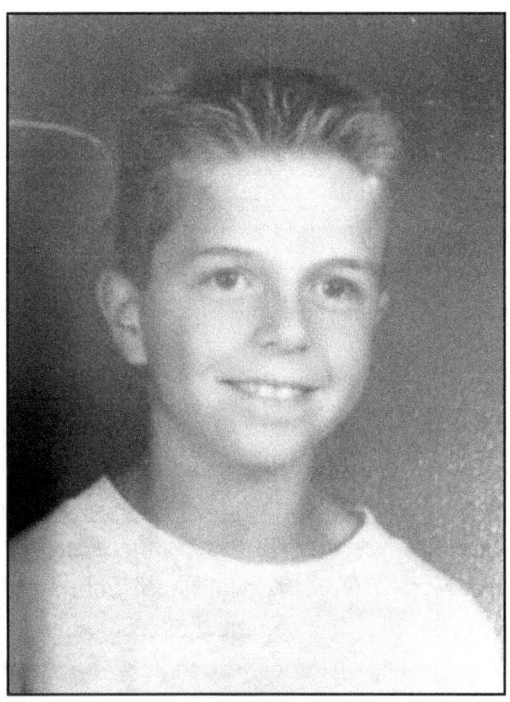

Dr. Williams

When I was eight years old, I had to have a tooth pulled. I remember it vividly—I was terrified! It started when I was staying with my grandmother while my parents were away on a work trip. I bit into something hard during a meal…crunch. There it was, a chunk of silver filling loose in my mouth. It didn't hurt, but I knew it was bad news. I had a gut-wrenching sensation in my stomach that every child feels when something is wrong. And I knew I'd have to visit the dentist when Mom and Dad got back in town. I wished their trip would have been longer…I hated going to any kind of doctor's office.

My nervousness grew when my parents returned, and my mom got on the phone to make the appointment. Her tone was serious, and she made the appointment for just a day or two away. Before I knew it, I was lying down with a bright light in my eyes, tears running down my checks as a needle poked into my gums. Suddenly, I had a "foot on my chest" as my dentist pushed my head back and forth, yanking on that broken baby tooth. While she did so, she talked to me, explaining that I needed to take better care of my teeth. She focused on flossing, saying that adding that one step would go a long way to protecting me from this—yank!—kind of—tug!—situation again.

When she was finally finished with her barbarian tactics, I got outta there— quick! I had no pain or problems after, and I became the best flosser the second grade had ever known, and I went more than twelve years from that day without another cavity. Though it was a brutal experience (thankfully, chair-side manner now is light-years ahead of where it was), I learned a good lesson.

Now I focus on pain-free, relaxed dentistry because I've been there and will never forget that experience. Kids and adults receive laughing gas or sedation whenever needed, so they don't have to experience archaic dentistry. Today, I am grateful because that life lesson taught me how to floss, and it helped me learn how to defend my adult teeth from all of the potentially harmful external influences for a lifetime. I'm also grateful that I've personally experienced both sides of the dentist chair, so I understand how much better comfortable dentistry is.

Brush

Brushing is the most common way we care for our teeth. You may forget to use mouthwash, you may hate to floss, but you most likely brush your teeth, if not twice a day, at least once. In fact, an MIT survey found that that Americans say a toothbrush is more important to them than their computers and cars. (I'll cite the study at the end of the book in case you want to offer a new toothbrush over a new car the next time your spouse or teenager asks.)

The Fascinating History of Brushes and Paste

We're far from the only ones to heap such praise on this deceptively simple invention. People have been brushing their teeth with some sort of tool since around 3500–3000 BCE. (Before that, it was the old "put a little toothpaste on the finger" trick, which some of us still practice when we realize we've forgotten to pack our toothbrush on a camping trip.) The first toothbrush was a twig chewed to have a frayed end. Chinese writings talk about pulling branches from good-smelling trees, probably to help with breath freshening. The miswak has been around for centuries and was used in Asia, the Middle East, and Africa. It is a therapeutic twig that comes from the *Salvadora persica* tree. It has medicinal properties and freshens breath while it cleans. You can still find them today. Later, toothbrushes were made from horsetail hair, bringing us closer to the modern toothbrush.

Toothbrushes went into mass production in 1780. You may be surprised by who their inventor was. William Addis decided he wanted to do something to improve upon teeth cleaners issued to British prisoners—because he himself was imprisoned! Then, prisons handed out what were basically rags to be used for this job. Addis drilled holes in a small animal bone, asked the guard for some bristles, and tied and glued those in place through the holes. Get this: after he got out of prison, he started a toothbrush business—in fact, the company, Wisdom, is still around (www.wisdom.com).

Toothpaste has as long a history as the toothbrush. Ancient Egyptians scrubbed their teeth with an abrasive powder made of ground-up oxen hooves, myrrh, eggshells, and pumice. Greeks and Romans used ground bones and shells. Everyone was focusing on grittiness to scour the gunk off their chompers. The Chinese, starting as early as 500 BCE, added flavoring like ginseng, herbs, and salt—mmm. Probably effective, but not the minty freshness I brushed with before my first date with the woman who's now my wife.

Thanks to these early innovators, we now have little excuse to avoid brushing. After thousands of years of fine-tuning, we have easy-to-use brushes that are found in a variety of stores, and some toothpaste tastes so good, I have to watch my kids, so they don't eat it.

Here are my three recommendations, which I call 2/2/20, on when and how long to brush:

1. Brush for 2 minutes.
2. Brush 2 times a day. (Brushing 3 times a day is OK, as long as you are soft on your gums—4 per day is probably overkill.)
3. Don't eat or drink for 20 minutes after brushing—let the important minerals coat your teeth for added protection.

———— ♦ ————

Brushing To-Dos
- *Hold your brush at a forty-five-degree angle against the gumline, angling toward the gums.*
- *Brush with tiny circles.*
- *Brush for at least two minutes each time. (For kids under*

age two, twice a day for one minute each time is usually sufficient because they have fewer teeth.) Use a stopwatch. Listen to your favorite two-minute song. Or if you're using an electric toothbrush, pay attention to its built-in timer. Many divide the two minutes into four thirty-second segments, one for each quarter of your mouth. When deciding how much time to spend brushing your teeth, the important thing to remember is that it's not about a prescribed amount of time—it's about cleaning all the surfaces of your teeth, front, back, and top. There are some great apps available for kids (and adults!) to make the two minutes more fun.

- Brush your tongue. That's where the germs that cause bad breath mostly live. I use a tongue scraper, which can be found at any pharmacy, or you can call my office, and I'll send you one with instructions on how to use it properly.

- Wait at least twenty minutes after eating before brushing. Brushing with toothpaste removes food remnants off your teeth and gums, but the second reason we use toothpaste is to coat our teeth with breath-freshening, enamel-saving minerals. When you eat, bacteria produce acid that temporarily weakens enamel. Brushing too soon after eating, especially after eating acidic foods, can easily damage enamel because it's in a weakened state.

- Instead of brushing right after eating, rinse your mouth out with water or chew xylitol gum to increase saliva production. These measures will help to wash away bacteria without damaging your teeth and will quickly bring your pH (acidity levels) closer to a neutral state. When our mouths spend too much time under the critical pH level, we are exponentially more susceptible to tooth decay, sensitivity, and oral disease. This is where soft drinks and energy drinks accelerate tooth decay. Water is the best dental insurance available today!

————•◆•————

Tools of the Trade

Modern toothbrushes and toothpastes are leaps and bounds above the horsehair-and-soot solution of yesteryear, but they're not all created equal. Here are some tips to review before you make your next purchase from the toothpaste aisle.

Choose the proper toothbrush. You should change your brush every few months. The ADA recommends buying a new toothbrush every three to four months. Over time, the bristles of a toothbrush wear down and become less effective at removing plaque and bacteria. It's also important to swap out your toothbrush after being sick; if you don't, the germs from your illness may reinfect you or someone you love. You're using your toothbrush to clean your teeth of dirt and "bugs" (bacteria), so some of those bad germs will linger in the wet bristles of your brush. You wash your towel every week or so, right? Same idea. Aerosols from toilet flushing have also been found on toothbrush bristles, so make sure you close the lid, and clean your toilet too! (Note: some newer electric brush models include a UV sanitizer that keeps bristles cleaner.) The first step in a cleaner mouth is a clean toothbrush. Here are some simple things to look for in a good toothbrush:

- Choose a toothbrush with soft bristles. Brushing with a hard-bristled toothbrush or using excessive force while brushing can slowly cause gums to recede, exposing the root of the tooth and leading to sensitivity. It is a tool to gently massage your gums, not to scrub or saw away at them.
- Choose a brush that you can maneuver around your mouth

easily. Toothbrush heads may be round or rectangular, bigger or smaller, on flexible necks or stiff ones. Ask yourself which one will work with the size of your mouth, the arrangement of your teeth, and how wide you can open your mouth.

- Go electric! Studies have shown manual brushes can do very well compared to high-grade electric ones, but it's tougher to be on point manually. I like the electric brush because you simply set it on each tooth rather than pushing. Some newer models also have sensors that shut off the brush if you push too hard.

Use toothpaste. Toothpaste has two important roles during brushing: (1) cleaning your teeth and (2) delivering important minerals to your teeth, such as calcium and fluoride and, from some pastes, natural supplements such as xylitol and aloe vera. These should remain undisturbed on teeth for twenty minutes after you brush, so they can coat, protect, and strengthen your smile. I brush for two minutes, two times per day, and then I avoid eating or drinking for twenty minutes so the minerals can strengthen my enamel and protect my gums. You don't want to wash the toothpaste's minerals off your teeth before they've penetrated the enamel safely. Remember the 2s: 2 minutes, 2 times per day, 20 minutes without food, drinks, or rinses.

Drink Water

Drinking water is the best drink for both mouth health—and overall health!

Our bodies are 60 percent water and are at our healthiest when we keep our water content high. Being hydrated means healthy nutrients are getting distributed throughout our bodies, our acidity levels are balanced, waste is being moved out, and muscles and joints are kept loose and limber.

The benefits are high for our mouths too. Teeth and gums contain high levels of water, so when mouths are properly hydrated, breath smell, swallowing ability, and mouth sensitivity improve. For example:

Water produces saliva, your first defense against tooth decay. Saliva is your ongoing natural cleaning source, washing away particles and naturally delivering calcium, fluoride, and phosphorus to your teeth. Dry mouth is a huge problem for seniors, as well as cancer patients, snoring and sleep apnea sufferers, and adults and children on various medications. Drinking water helps offset some of the problems with dry mouth. For more dry mouth tips, see the dry mouth section in this book—it's a huge problem for our teeth and diet in today's world.

Water cleans with every sip. It washes away leftover food before it can get lodged between your teeth and under your gums and begin the process of decay. It also buffers and dilutes the acids produced by bacteria found in your mouth. By contrast, other drinks, including juice, leave things behind, like sugar and acids. These eat away at your teeth and feed your mouth's bacteria, which causes cavities.

Research shows that every time we sip an acidic beverage (including juices, diet drinks, and sports drinks), acid coats our teeth for thirty to sixty minutes. Heartburn and acid reflux have the same damaging effects on teeth as soft drinks do. So, if you brush your teeth two times per day for two minutes each but drink two sodas per day, you are losing a mouth marathon at a rate of four minutes of cleaning versus two hours of acidic damage. That's an uphill battle!

It's important to recognize energy drinks as popular beverages that are causing growing dental disease -- I treat rotted teeth, requiring costly root canals almost every day. Most people have long accepted that sodas are dangerous because of the sugar; more recently, people are realizing that fruit juices are not a healthy alternative to soft drinks but are nearly as sugary and bad for teeth. (Juice has been shown to have zero nutritional value.) Energy drinks now are causing concern, hiding under the guise of being "healthy" or for active adults "on the go." Kids and teens guzzle them after sports practices, with meals, and to give them a supposed extra boost to get through classes. Researchers have found that the drinks' high levels of citric acid, malic acid, and/or phosphoric, added for improved flavor and shelf life, strip teeth of their enamel (which is designed by nature to protect teeth from decay). Beverage companies aren't required to declare on product labels the amount of citric acid they contain. "No sugar" diet drinks are proving to be very harmful on teeth as well, due to the many preservatives and acids. Studies have shown diet drinks may be just as likely to cause insulin problems in people with diabetes as regular sugar sodas are.

———◆———

What's at Stake
About 13 percent of adolescents ages twelve to nineteen in the United States have at least one untreated decayed tooth; that number jumps to 20 percent for children ages five to eleven. According to CDC reports, fluoridated water is one of the best ways to combat tooth decay. In fact, for every one dollar spent in prevention, such as fluoridated water, up to thirty-eight dollars are saved in future dental treatment costs. That's a 3800% savings!

———◆———

Hidden Popsicles: Judson's First Lesson in Oral Health

Sugary and acidic drinks are not the only culprits causing adolescent and childhood tooth decay. Sour candy, bread, crackers, and chips leave similarly destructive starches and preservatives on our teeth for minutes or even hours after we consume them.

One summer when my son, Judson, was about four years old, he began a sneaky habit. He would wake up before his mom and me and sneak out back to eat popsicles. He was quiet about it too. He would carefully shut the screen door to the back porch and would even throw his wrappers away. Eventually we caught him when we found a mountain of Otter Pop wrappers in the garbage can outside. A few months later, I found his first cavity on an X-ray—and it was huge! Even with Dental Dad helping him brush and floss daily, he nearly lost a baby tooth that he needed to keep for at least six more years for proper jaw and teeth development.

————— • ◆ • —————

Water contains fluoride, in most cities in the United States. Tooth decay was on the rise until water fluoridation began in the 1945, with Grand Rapids, Michigan, being the first city to fluoridate. Then, for several decades, tooth decay was decreasing, up until sugary drinks and sodas began to dramatically rise in consumption.

Fluoride is considered "nature's natural cavity fighter" because it occurs naturally in many foods, as well as water, and protects teeth from cavity-causing bacteria. Bacteria that are in plaque produce acids that adhere to and break down our protective enamel. Fluoride makes tooth enamel more resistant to bacteria's acid attacks by combining with the phosphorus and calcium in our saliva to form an even stronger and smoother mineral coating than nature gave us.

The key to safety and efficacy is the level of fluoridation in water:

under one part per million is considered a safe level. That's less than one drop of fluoride for every 1 million drops of water. Occasionally I will meet a patient with brown pits or rough pits on their teeth from drinking well water in rural areas. Well water may have concentrations of fluoride of six parts per million or more—six times or more than the recommended dosage. This is considered too high and not recommended by professionals. Most bottled water and many fridge-filtered waters do not contain fluoride. So I'll continue to give my kids tap water until they are twelve to thirteen years old and all of their teeth are erupted. If used correctly, fluoridated water can be a huge help, especially for developing teens and children.

The Science Behind Fluoride

Here's why fluoride works so well with our teeth. Hydroxyapatite is a strong, naturally occurring crystal-like mineral form of calcium and fluoride found in our teeth and bones. Hydroxyapatite is found elsewhere in nature as well, such as in sea coral. Fluorhydroxyapatite is hydroxyapatite combined with fluoride to make a super-strong mineral shell on teeth. So, when this important mineral (fluoride) is used properly, teeth can become stronger and whiter.

Think of a natural tooth as being like a stone: smooth, strong, and resistant to invasion. When you consume high levels of starches, acidic drinks, sweets or are malnourished, the stone begins to weaken and become porous. For many who drink high levels of soft drinks, their teeth begin to look like volcanic rock—much weaker and more brittle, plus the pores can grow larger and are open to invasion. When we correctly apply fluoride to the rock (tooth) in time, it takes on the good properties of hydroxyapatite and makes the teeth even stronger. The strengthened enamel looks more like granite or quartz than volcanic rock—smoother, harder, and more resistant to invasion.

Fluoride helps repair tooth decay in its earliest stages by building up the tooth in a process called remineralization. Remineralization is when hydroxyapatite can transform into fluorhydroxyapatite. This cavity-fighting mineral even reduces the ability of plaque bacteria to produce acid in the first place. It can arrest the plaque and push the "pause button" on it before it breaks into our teeth. Truly, fluoride is the best natural cavity fighter out there, helping our teeth stay healthy and strong. Xylitol sugar is not only great for our teeth and sinus, but it has been shown to give fluoride a natural boost (more on xylitol later in this book). These changes aren't usually visual to the human eye, but they are visible under a microscope. You can feel the improvements with less sensitivity, fewer cavities, and more successful checkups.

Exposure to fluoride can be especially beneficial for infants and children. For kids between the ages of six months and sixteen years, fluoride becomes incorporated into developing permanent teeth, protecting them from cavity-causing bacteria. The ADA and the CDC have reported that children who drink fluoridated tap water have fewer decayed teeth than those who do not. Simply by drinking water, a person receives fluoride's protective benefits.

There is a vocal minority who disagree with fluoride being added to water. They cite studies that point to negative effects of ingesting fluoride regularly, but those studies are fewer and less convincing than those supporting it.

If everyone used fluoridated toothpaste properly, consumed fewer sugar drinks and starchy foods, drank more water, and received fluoride treatments regularly at the dentist, we may not need fluoride in the water. But until that happens, adding the naturally occurring mineral to the water serves the general population well, especially underserved, high-risk, and malnourished populations. Why take the risk?

———◆———

The Drink Challenge

Because I've always been intrigued by teeth and I'm a bit of a science nerd, I saved my wisdom teeth after they were removed when I was a teenager. (Interestingly, I've never had a patient tell me they kept their wisdom teeth after having them removed…) Years later, after dental school, I finally decided what to do with them: have my teeth become my own research project.

More and more of my patients were suffering from broken and decayed teeth due to poor diet and consuming soft drinks. I decided to test just how quickly some popular soft drinks could destroy my wisdom teeth, which were healthy and cavity-free when they were removed. Like many people, I had wisdom teeth that were coming in crooked, were hard to reach and clean, and were likely to negatively impact my other teeth. I was also leaving the country for some volunteer work for my church, and I didn't want to have any issues while I was away. So my dentist and parents decided it was best to remove them. I have never missed them, nor did it lessen my ability to chew and eat.

I placed each one of my four pearly whites into a glass of each of the following drinks: Coca-Cola, G2 (low-calorie) Gatorade, Mountain Dew, and Diet Coke. The drinks damaged my teeth from worst to least in that order, but the difference among them was slight. In less than a week, all four teeth looked like sponges when placed under a microscope. The enamel had been destroyed, leaving chalky and brittle teeth behind. Under a microscope, they went from looking like smooth, hard glass to porous sponges. Within just a few days, the clear liquid beverages were turned cloudy with all of the mineral content that had leached out of my teeth. Trying to justify why Diet Coke is less harmful on our teeth than regular Coke is like saying washing a car every eleven months is better than washing it once a year.

It offers only the barest of improvement. To see photos of my experiment, see the resources section of this book.

———◆———

Use Xylitol

Xylitol is a great natural sugar alternative that not only satisfies your craving for sweet things but even supports oral and sinus health. Start your kids off right—buy them some sugar-free, xylitol-sweetened gum, suckers, or mints and encourage them to use them after eating or in place of sugary snacks. It's also safe and helpful for nursing and pregnant mothers. This natural sweetener is even perfect for people with diabetes because it metabolizes without using insulin. In my home, we often use xylitol sugar granules in place of table sugar for sweetening fruit, making smoothies and ice cream, and baking. See the resources section of this book if you'd like me to send you a free sample of some xylitol mints or candies.

The History of Xylitol

Xylitol was born out of a sugar shortage in Finland, during World War II. Desperate for a sweet alternative, the Finnish people started harvesting xylitol from their birch forests. About thirty years later, researchers discovered that xylitol safely arrests the mouth bacteria that causes tooth decay.

Finland has had an official preventative health care program since 1972. This means restoring dental problems is a secondary objective, not the primary health plan. This is now the standard of care for modern dentistry. In 2013, the Finnish National Institute of Health & Welfare recommended that all one-to-six-year-olds be given xylitol after meals.

That same year, the Ministry of Social Affairs and Health also recommended that xylitol products be used to improve dental health and to decrease the costs of dental care. The results have been impressive, not only in improving the health of children and adults but in bringing awareness to this helpful natural derivative.

Two of my favorite companies that make various xylitol products are Xlear (www.xlear.com) and Branam Healthy Smiles for Life (www.branamsmile.com). They make various mints, gums, mouth rinse, toothpastes, and sweeteners that not only taste great but are much better for you than table sugar or artificial sweeteners. For my highest-risk patients, or those who suffer with severe dry mouth, we use Carifree prescription products (www.carifree.com), which are available through select dental professionals.

Conclusion

With proper and regular flossing and brushing, as well as good habits like drinking water and replacing sugar with alternatives like xylitol, you can have a healthy mouth and avoid a lot of expensive, painful corrective procedures. Simply focus on preventative measures to avoid expensive dental treatments later. There's a myth that has crept into the thoughts of many people: that caring for teeth is expensive, time consuming, and uncomfortable and that teeth are too much work to maintain or save. Before I became a dentist, I thought some people just had "bad" or "soft" teeth. But this thinking is wrong and unhelpful for those in need. It just isn't true! Preventative care costs less per month than a cable bill or cell phone plan, usually much less. For such little effort and money, you can avoid most major dental work, and you'll improve your total-body health in the process.

THREE

The Mouth, the Gateway to the Body

As I mentioned in the previous chapter on simple and cost-effective ways to greatly minimize unnecessary trips to the dentist, there are reasons to keep your mouth healthy beyond the borders of your lips. Oral health equals whole-body health. Conversely, if you're not paying attention to your teeth and gums, you could find yourself making a trip to the doctor or surgeon, as well as the dentist. Studies have found links between mouth health and multiple diseases that occur elsewhere in the body. They've also shown that overall health issues can lead to poor oral health. All organs and systems in our body are tightly interconnected and serve as warning signs to alert us to something that is changing or worsening. With proper, immediate attention, we can make our bodies whole when we focus on the oral-systemic balance.

Diabetes

Diabetes and poor oral health sync in multiple ways: Symptoms of diabetes can be seen in the mouth. Diabetes damages dental health. Periodontal care can improve diabetes care, especially for those who have uncontrolled or fluctuating blood sugar levels. In fact, many diabetic patients have gum disease and vice versa. Those with either unmanaged gum disease or uncontrolled diabetes are at a much higher risk for other diseases as well as losing their teeth and ability to eat properly.

As of 2017, nearly 30 million people in the United States are affected by diabetes, and approximately 1.7 million new people are being diagnosed each year. The disease affects the body's ability to process sugar. Because the body converts food into sugar to be used as energy, any malfunction in this is problematic, affects qualify of life, and can even be fatal.

Early signs of diabetes include feeling incredibly thirsty. This is in part because diabetes can lower a person's ability to produce saliva. Without enough saliva, teeth are threatened in their first defense against cavities. Combined with the body's weakening resistance to infection, gums may become inflamed, bleed, and develop disease.

Twenty-two percent of people with diabetes have gum disease, or periodontal disease. The number is much higher for adults over age sixty-five, jumping up to more than 70 percent. Poor blood sugar control in those with diabetes creates an environment in which bad bacteria living in the mouth can grow stronger and attack the gums and jawbones. The bacteria progressively break down the protective supportive tissues holding the teeth until they get too lose or too hard to maintain and are lost. Unmanaged gum disease is the number one reason adults lose their teeth. In turn, this infection may cause blood sugar to rise, which a person with diabetes has a hard time fighting, which continues the vicious circle between diabetes and periodontal disease.

One symptom of diabetes is poor blood circulation. Our mouths are red inside because there's so much blood flow needed to keep it healthy. Poor circulation leads to poor oxygen levels in these areas of our bodies. No oxygen—no life! This why people with diabetes have such a high rate of early tooth loss.

However, there's also a positive relationship between the two diseases. Improving the health of gums through preventative, home care, and/or minor surgical procedures can improve blood sugar control, actually slowing diabetes' progression. According to research reported by the ADA, home care of teeth and gums (that is, primarily, flossing, brushing, eating right, and drinking water) as well as regular cleaning and maintenance at the dentist can improve a person's HbA1c. (An HbA1c is a blood-based lab test that shows how well diabetes is controlled.) Keeping this within a safe range ensures patients are healthy enough to have routine treatment without concerns for diabetic shock or unstable blood sugar levels.

Heart Disease

Stroke. Heart attack. Hardening of arteries. Periodontitis. Cavities. Oral health is proven to be linked to heart disease. People with poor oral health are at an increased risk for heart disease over those with healthy mouths. The growth of artery plaque is an inflammatory process, as is the progression of gum disease—and more and more research is connecting the two.

For example, endocarditis, an infection of the heart's inner lining, is caused by bacteria traveling through the bloodstream and attaching to the heart. That bacteria can come from the mouth. Mouth bacteria migrating into the bloodstream can also cause elevated C-reactive protein, which inflames blood vessels and leads to stroke.

I watched a documentary about the story of a preacher who nearly lost his life from a tooth infection. His doctors could find nothing wrong with him. Countless tests were of no help. Finally, one of his physicians suggested he see a dentist because he hadn't in some time. A panoramic dental X-ray showed several infected teeth—which were determined as the cause of his nearly fatal illness. The teeth had no symptoms. Totally painless, but they nearly took his life! See the resources section of this book for a link to the documentary.

According to experts in the *Journal of Periodontology* and the *American Journal of Cardiology*, a consensus could soon be reached between the two fields of medicine: heart health and oral health. WebMD reported on the work in 2009. From a review of 120 studies, papers, and other data, they concluded:

- Periodontal disease is a risk factor for coronary artery disease. Families of certain bacteria found in gum and heart diseases are the same.
- A high level of C-reactive protein is common in both people with gum disease and those with heart disease. This protein level measures the level of inflammation in our bodies. Inflammation has been shown to lead to chronic disease and a lower quality of life.

The evidence between the two types of diseases is strong enough for there to be a bigger push for dentists to talk with patients about heart problems if those patients have moderate to severe gum disease. Doctors with patients with at-risk hearts should suggest they visit a periodontist. In the future, physicians and dentists will better work together to support reducing gum and heart risk. In the future, dentists will likely administer painless screenings to test for diabetes at a routine dental checkup, saving time, money, and health for everyone. We are working to make the future of prevention happen now.

Pregnancy Issues

Poor dental health can negatively affect unborn babies and their mothers. The lesser-known secret lies in the fact that pregnancy changes the body in more ways than just growing a baby. Those changes can cause oral health issues, which can negatively affect the unborn baby. A pregnant body requires more blood flow, requires more calcium, and produces more hormones, all of which can cause problems in the mouth if not addressed early.

———◆———

A Very Personal Connection Made
Between Pregnancy and Dentistry

While I was a first-year dental student, my wife, Megan, and I were blessed to find out that she was pregnant with our first child, Judson. We also learned the effects pregnancy can have on the oral environment.

One day, while I was carving teeth out of wax in my anatomy lab, I received a call for help from Megan. She had incredible mouth pain and was scared. She didn't know what to do—she'd never experienced pain like this before. We got her into the emergency dental clinic quickly. We found a retained baby tooth in her mouth. An adult tooth had never grown in, and therefore she still had a baby molar. These teeth are designed to make space for our adult teeth and growing jaw during adolescence, but they have small, thin roots and aren't designed to last into adulthood. A pain-relieving filling was put into the tooth, and Megan was put on pregnancy-safe antibiotics, and she recovered just fine.

A few months after our bundle of joy arrived, Megan was in the student dental clinic as my patient for her scheduled checkup. (I thank her for helping me pass a few of my requirements to graduate!) Upon reviewing routine X-rays and an evaluation, we learned she had more than six new cavities! She was shocked! She generally practiced great home mouth care. The answer, to why the baby tooth had made its presence known and why there was an upswing in number of cavities, was simple and singular: pregnancy. Pregnancy has a dramatic effect on the mother's teeth, oral environment, and of course, other areas of the body.

———◆———

The reasons for increased risk of decay and gum disease during pregnancy vary but include: fluctuating hormone levels (such as estrogen and progesterone), changes in diet, calcium needs of the body, and dry mouth. Here are seven things to remember when you or a loved one are pregnant:

1. Gum disease: During pregnancy and maternity, the mother's gums require special attention to stay healthy. Regular brushing and flossing are great, but also eating a balanced diet and visiting the dentist twice during pregnancy for checkups and gum evaluation will help prevent or reduce pregnancy-related issues. Studies suggest that gum disease triggers increased levels of labor-inducing biological fluids. There's also research linking low birth weight (under five pounds, eight ounces) and premature delivery (less than thirty-seven weeks) and gum disease.

2. Periodontal disease and diabetes: Periodontitis has been documented to cause infertility in couples where one or both partner is affected. Gum disease may be temporary during pregnancy, called pregnancy gingivitis, but it can become permanent if not addressed. It's similar to gestational diabetes in pregnant mothers, which can become long-term diabetes if Mom doesn't stay healthy during and after pregnancy.

3. Swellings and growths: Pregnancy tumors can cause discomfort, excess bleeding, or sensitivity. They are lumps along the gums caused by plaque and changes in hormones. They usually go away on their own, or minor surgery can remove them if they are uncomfortable.

4. Enamel erosion: Morning sickness and nausea can cause excess vomiting that attacks enamel. Rinsing vigorously with water after vomiting and using a fluoride rinse in the morning help protect teeth.

5. Dry mouth: Pregnancy-induced dry mouth will increase risks for tooth decay and sensitivity, as well as infections. A pregnant woman should drink lots of water each day (which is good for

the baby anyway!) and chew a sugarless gum to increase saliva flow and remove food particles from your teeth. Plus, it may help distract her nose if she is experiencing a heightened sense of smell during pregnancy.

6. It's safe to visit the dentist: I've been asked this question more times than I can count. There's some old myth that you can't see the dentist if you are pregnant or that you can't have procedures done. While we always use precaution and a riskbased assessment, I've never had a problem or complication with treating my pregnant patients. Cleanings, cavity fillings, root canals, and even tooth removal are just fine. X-rays are safe if needed, especially if they are digital, which has an incredibly low dose of radiation—less than being in the sun for a few hours.

7. Sedatives: Laughing gas is not recommended, but sedatives can be used if Mom is in a high level of pain. Typically, we administer a safe dose of local anesthesia, and the procedures go great, as long as we remember Mom may have some discomfort from sitting for long periods, depending on which trimester she is in. We can help that with cushions or blankets and keeping appointments shorter as needed.

We can help with cushions or blankets and keeping appointments short.

Recently, I removed two wisdom teeth from one of my pregnant patients, and she did great! Her wisdom teeth were decayed, and we decided that the risk of leaving her decay and gingivitis around the wisdom teeth, was much higher than the risk of the routine procedure. She had really bad breath from a lack of cleaning for several years, multiple cavities, and gum swelling around her wisdom teeth. We broke it up into two appointments, first her evaluation and cleaning and then second a visit for her procedures. Local anesthetic was administered, and she was done in under eight minutes. Multiple teeth had the decay removed and were restored with boned fillings. The wisdom teeth came out without any issues, and she had almost no bleeding. She was happy to have it done, and her baby was still on track to be delivered in a few more months. I followed up with her a week later, and both she and her partner were amazed at how quickly she recovered, and that she was eating her regular diet by the next day!

Fortunately, there is lot that can be done to prevent or correct oral issues even during pregnancy. You should continue your home health care routine of flossing and brushing. You should still use antigingivitis mouthwash and fluoride toothpaste. Annual exams and preventive dental care during pregnancy are not only safe but recommended. As soon as you find out you're pregnant, you can make an appointment to talk with your dentist for help preventing common pregnancy-related dental concerns. Even X-rays, medications, and anesthetics can be used as needed—just let your dentist know about your pregnancy, so any risks are known and weighed. Contrary to popular belief, new technology allows for pregnant mothers to safely have cavities and gum disease treated during pregnancy. Digital X-rays are very safe and have an incredibly low amount of radiation. In fact, a four-hour plane flight has as much radiation as over one hundred standard digital periapical X-rays. Plus, we can take intraoral photos with a small and specialized mouth camera—these digital pictures of your mouth allow you to see what we see. Modern dentistry allows a mother and baby to feel safe and healthy during pregnancy.

Diseases of Age

As the body changes with time, other connections between oral health and overall health can be drawn.

Osteoporosis, which affects more than 53 million people in the United States alone, can affect the jawbone. This disease makes bones less dense, so the jaw holding the teeth may be affected. Periodontal disease becomes more common. Studies have shown that women with osteoporosis are three times more likely to experience tooth loss than people who don't have the disease.

People with Alzheimer's and dementia can also struggle with oral health. This is in part because these patients will experience ever decreasing mental capacity to care for themselves. Having a consistent, ingrained home care habit before the diagnosis can help patients maintain it longer. Beyond that, there may be a connection between illnesses of the mind and those of the mouth. As it is in so many cases, that connection may involve inflammation. Inflammation has been linked to many diseases, including those also related to aging, such as stroke, Alzheimer's, and heart disease.

Malnutrition

Poor diet and unhealthy mouths go hand in hand. Highly processed foods (like those that come in boxes, cans, and wrappers) contain more sugars, preservatives, and acids than whole foods (fresh fruits and veggies, whole grains, and eggs). Eating processed foods negatively affects oral health and the major organs and blood vessels in the body. These foods are less nutritious than whole foods, leaving the body's defenses less equipped to resist and fight infection. This leads to accelerated tooth loss, which perpetuates the malnutrition problem—a person with weaker or fewer teeth can't easily eat apples or carrots. Foods must then be soft, which likely means starchy and processed, and therefore full of simple, acid-inducing sugars.

This was a major problem where I spent time on rotations in dental school, in south and southwest Virginia. It is an incredibly beautiful part of our country, with rolling green hills, fresh air, and beautiful views. But rates of high blood pressure and diabetes in this area are high for this very reason. It is one of the most challenged areas of the country (at the time of this writing) for dental health. Some people drive for hours to reach a dentist or doctor. Plus, the education on nutrition and health has not been well developed. Multiple times we removed most or all remaining teeth on people younger than me, and I was only twenty-nine years old at the time! Fortunately, the dental school I attended and the Commonwealth of Virginia have given a lot of resources to this area, often in the form of MOM Projects—Missions of Mercy, donations and fundraisers. As part of the MOM Projects, student dentists treat hundreds, and sometimes thousands, of patients for little or no cost to them. It was one of the most memorable experiences of dental school for me, and it is changing the outlook of whole communities on dentistry and health, bringing awareness and better access to care.

Conclusion

While there are many more studies underway to better link oral health and systemic health, most experts agree that there is a strong connection—because the mouth is the gateway of the body. Any improvement or degradation of one part will affect and be affected by others.

The good news I can leave you with is that if the negative aspects are interconnected, so are the positive. Getting your whole body in shape and staying that way will help your mouth's health as much as it will help your heart, lungs, brain, and digestive system health. Just like with diet and exercise, the key isn't just to get healthy but to work daily on staying that way. It's a marathon, not a sprint.

FOUR

Dry Mouth: The Hidden Threat to Millions of Adults

There are four big challenges for oral health in adults. They are:

1. Tooth decay (the most commonly known oral disease)

2. Periodontal disease (the number one reason for adult tooth loss)

3. Oral cancer (on the rise in nonsmokers, teens, and adults)

4. Dry mouth, or xerostomia

5. Sleep apnea and/or teeth grinding

In this chapter, I discuss silent threat number four: dry mouth. The biggest issue I've found with dry mouth is that most people don't know or aren't warned about the harm it causes to our teeth. I've had and currently have many patients who have suffered silently from dry mouth. Many have lost multiple teeth, even though they were brushing and flossing at home. They thought they were doing all the right things, yet still something clearly went wrong. Aside from severely weakened teeth, dry mouth also makes us feel thirsty more often, increases teeth sensitivity, makes saliva thick or clumpy, creates an unpleasant film at the corners of our lips, and makes it tougher to eat, chew, and swallow.

Causes of Dry Mouth

Dry mouth is usually caused by at least one of three factors: mouth breathing, medications, radiation, or cancer treatments. Mouth breathing is common in adults and children and can be due to any of the following: development of a high palate with narrow jaws, large tonsils or small airway, nasal septum blockage, TMJ or teeth grinding, or sleep apnea. Cancer treatments such as radiation shrink or destroy important saliva ducts and glands in the head and neck, leaving teeth and gums vulnerable. Saliva contains important minerals to help strengthen the teeth, as well as enzymes to help us digest and swallow our food. When saliva flow is decreased, starches and foods stick to the teeth longer, which are already more vulnerable from lower mineral exposure, creating a negative feedback loop—unless action is taken.

In my practice, medication-induced dry mouth is the most common cause of xerostomia. Recently, I obtained a twenty-three-page print-out of common medications that cause dry mouth. You probably have several dry-mouth-inducing medications in your own kitchen cabinet right now, so beware! Common medications (both prescription and nonprescription, as reported by the Mayo Clinic) that cause or increase dry mouth are drugs prescribed to address:

- Asthma or breathing problems (this is one of the most common categories I see, especially from steroid inhalers)
- Depression
- Pain, soreness, or muscle spasms
- Nausea and dizziness
- Allergies
- Anxiety
- Acne and other skin issues
- High blood pressure
- Colds
- Weight control
- Urinary incontinence

If you regularly take medications for any of these reasons, I urge you to read the labels and talk to your doctor and dentist. Many people don't notice symptoms of dry mouth until it's too late: teeth began to decay at the gumline, root canals fail, and enamel breaks and chips. Then they wonder, "Why is this happening? I brush my teeth every day!" It is tough for me to see a patient's smile decay from this silent threat. It must be even tougher for the patient to go through this frustrating condition.

Treatment of Dry Mouth

If you have even the slightest amount of dry mouth, there are some great things you can do to strengthen your enamel. Drinking water when you are thirsty isn't enough. Going to the dentist twice a year isn't enough. Brushing twice a day and flossing once a day aren't enough. But using multiple techniques does work well. Here are my six tips to dramatically reduce dry mouth damage to your teeth.

1. Drink water after every meal or snack.

2. Ensure you have the proper amount of calcium in your diet.

3. Avoid diet drinks and sodas; the acid will amplify the effects of dry mouth.

4. Strive for five: five exposures per day to xylitol, that is. Gums, mints, and candies are great. There are also some wonderful slow-release xylitol discs that adhere to your cheek or roof of your mouth and slowly dissolve while you sleep (e.g., Xylimelts by Oracoat). These time-release lozenges are a tremendous help for my sleep apnea patients and dry mouth patients.

5. Get a fluoride varnish application at your dentist three to four times per year. It is more than twenty-two times stronger than regular toothpaste, reduces sensitivity, and is very safe because

it is applied topically. I don't suffer with dry mouth, but genetic gum recession runs in my family, so I have the varnish applied Dry Mouth: The Hidden Threat to Millions of Adults ... 59 ... to my teeth four times per year. The latest research shows fluoride varnish provides three to six months of benefits. Drinking water just doesn't cut it in developed adults (age sixteen and older). Over-the-counter toothpaste is more than 1,000 times stronger than drinking water. Varnish is 2,200 times more powerful than over-the-counter toothpaste.

6. Use a professional-grade electric toothbrush, which will clean much better around your crowns, fillings, implants, and retainers. It will sweep away the plaque much quicker and more thoroughly than a manual brush will for most people.

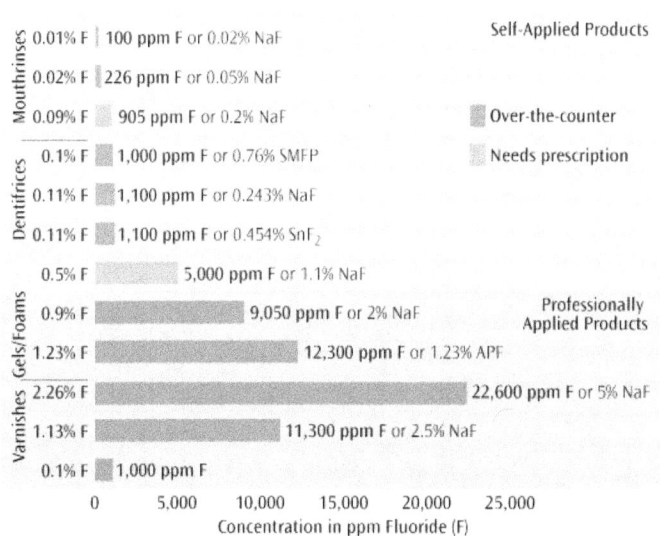

By following these steps, or sharing them with someone who suffers from dry mouth, you can save more teeth, avoid frustration, and have better breath and healthier, sensitivity-free gums. I hope more pharmaceutical and medical awareness will be paid to these powerful side effects in medications. Medications are important, and often life-saving. We need them. But we can do more to protect our oral health by staying informed and ahead of the ball.

FIVE

Aging Population: The Oral Health Secrets to Living Longer!

We are living longer than ever! This is the result of healthier diets, improved technology, longer work careers, and most importantly, better awareness of our health. When social security was designed, the average life expectancy was under sixty-two years of age. Now it's closer to eighty years of age—a 29 percent increase in life expectancy. Baby boomers are a unique generation in that they are the first to have the opportunity to save or replace all of their natural teeth and are the first generation to see the dentist regularly for checkups. Their parents also visited the dentist in adulthood, but as kids in the early 1900s, most parents of baby boomers did not see the dentist unless there was an emergency or a toothache. Longer lifespans are fantastic, but it's created some difficulties for those who live longer. Often, older people are on a fixed income and need advanced dental care, which is rarely, if ever, covered by basic dental insurance or Medicare.

Here are six commonplace oral health challenges affecting our aging population:

1. Sleep apnea

2. TMJ and "bruxism" (teeth grinding)

3. Heartburn and acid reflux

4. Medications and dry mouth

5. Periodontal disease

6. Oral cancer

The "Bruxism Triad"

Sleep apnea effects not only our total health, but our mouths. Every year many lives are taken from sleep apnea. Often sleep apnea is paired with "bruxism" or nighttime teeth grinding. Pair these two with acid reflux or heartburn and we have what is known at the "The Bruxism Triad."

I first learned of this back in 2010 from research done by Dr. Jeffrey Rouse. His findings studied the association between grinding, sleep apnea and acid reflux. I have been a follower of this science ever since I learned of the association, and I have reated many of my own patients with these conditions since then.

———•———

Avoid the Daily Grind!

What is that terrible noise? Not long after my beautiful wife, Megan, and I were married, I awoke one night to a terrible sound. Was someone breaking into the house? Was something outside rattling in the wind? Was the air conditioner squeaking?

It turned out that Megan was a nighttime "bruxer." Bruxism is a disorder caused by teeth grinding. Even though I'm a heavy sleeper, my "dentist sense" alerts me to such things! She never complained of headaches, sore jaws, or teeth, but her parents had known—or heard—that something was happening in her sleep, and it needed to be corrected. They had taken her to the dentist regularly when she was a child and teen, but no one had ever given her a solution for her teeth grinding. Later, her college roommates reminded Megan that this disturbing gnashing of teeth was still happening. Time passed. Her roommates put in earplugs. She was young and otherwise healthy, so grinding hadn't affected her smile too much at this point (at least not to the casual eye). I now wasn't going to let her beautifully beaming smile be ruined!

Fortunately, when we got married and her nighttime noises first woke me, I had just begun my training in dental school, so I had an idea of what was going on and that we could do something about it. In fact, we had to, for the sake of her mouth health, not just to keep me from having dental nightmares. At our dental clinic, we learned she had multiple teeth that were wearing down prematurely and several tooth fillings that had chips, gaps, and wear on them. Her risk for tooth decay and yellowed teeth was greatly increased by these problems.

Megan's complete treatment plan included conservative bonding of her worn teeth, replacement of worn fillings, and a night guard to wear during sleep. Since Megan has started wearing a night guard, it has been years since she has chipped a tooth or worn out a filling prematurely. She is good about wearing it regularly, and you can really see the wear on the guard, which is much better than wear chiseling down her teeth like it used to.

I find that one-third to one-half of my adult patients have a history of teeth grinding, usually without knowing it. Studies have confirmed this is an accurate range, and that teeth wear up to ten times faster when someone is bruxing or clenching! Think *of a table leg: It's great at supporting a force or load verti-cally, from the top down. A well-made table or chair can usually handle several hundred pounds when used correctly. However, it you come at that leg sideways, it can really shorten the life of the table.*

It's always eye-opening for my patients who get a custom guard to see the scratches and wear on those dental appliances. This is so much better than wear on teeth, because although durable and made to last years, guards are replaceable, but natural teeth are not. Some of my patients don't believe it, until after just a few days or weeks wearing an appliance, and it looks like someone took it off-road in the Uinta Mountains. It really is amazing to see what can happen, often unknowingly, to our teeth!

Dry Mouth

Dry mouth was discussed in some length earlier in this book, but it has become such a huge concern for adults that I want to mention it again in the context of older adults. Many people view tooth decay as some-thing that only happens to kids who eat treats and don't brush before bed. The truth is, for dry mouth sufferers, brush and flossing alone are not enough. By using the home techniques discussed in this book and scheduling more frequent visits to the dentist, older people can avoid early tooth loss or unnecessary dental procedures.

In the last year or two of my grandfather's life, he experienced ex-treme dry mouth coupled with dementia and poor home hygiene. The teeth he took such great of for so many years were lost quickly. His bridges didn't fit anymore, so his ability to chew was hampered im-mensely. He didn't complain much about his teeth because he wasn't the complaining type. But he was very frustrated with his inability to chew. Every month he was losing more teeth. It was heartbreaking for the family, plus it made his eating habits worse since he ate more snacks and processed foods that he didn't touch when he was healthy.

Periodontal Disease

Periodontal disease is on the rise. Simply put, if you live longer, you have more risks for tooth loss. It's kind of like owning a car. Part of vehicle ownership is maintenance, and as our vehicles (or mouths) put on more miles every year, they need even more upkeep to run smoothly and reliably.

Wisdom teeth pose a high risk for gum disease in many adults. It is still up for debate whether wisdom teeth cause other teeth to crowd or shift over time. One thing I know for sure is so many adults have a hard time cleaning around those teeth way back there and usually cannot or do not floss adequately. As a result, we see a high rate of gingivitis or periodontitis in third molars (the dental term for wisdom teeth).

Most people elect to have wisdom teeth removed for this very reason; plus, maintaining them over time or having them bonded, crowned, or treated for root canal infection is more costly than having them re-moved. If you are considering having yours removed, the younger you are the better, but I've routinely removed them in patients as old as eighties and nineties without complication. If you cannot commit to a high level of home care, talk to your dentist about removal, even if you are older. Today, most people heal very quickly, and not having wisdom teeth does not impair the ability to chew. I've never had a patient tell me they missed their wisdom tooth after having them removed.

While you get your next checkup, ask to have a periodontal mapping, a measured charting of your gums and their pockets. If they are 3mm and under, you are considered low-risk for gum disease, and regular checkups two times per year may be all you need going forward. If they measure at 4mm or higher, you may need additional therapy or periodontal care to get back to health.

With increased preparation and care, we can expect extra high-quality years of eating, speaking, and smiling with confidence. You don't have to suffer with gradual tooth loss, bad breath, sensitive teeth, and decreased ability to chew if you take early action. Today we have great less invasive options to make gums and jawbone healthier, and more comfortably than ever!

Oral Cancer

Oral cancer is a huge threat, especially in those who have a family history of cancer, are exposed to the human papillomavirus (HPV), drink alcohol, smoke or chew, or wear dentures or removable partial dentures. When detected and addressed in early stages, it is very treatable and has minimal, if any, impact on quality of life. When found in stage three or stage four, however, the recurrence rate is high and often fatal within just a few years.

If you haven't already, get to a dentist this year. When you are there, ask what preventative services are offered. Get your annual oral cancer screening—it is painless and easier than ever. Ask about digital technology, such as intraoral cameras and digital X-rays, so you can see what your dentist and hygienist see. Dentistry costs pennies on the dollar compared to most medical expenses, and you'll be so much better informed going forward.

Conclusion

Aging adults have many options to preserve a bright smile, and the earlier you act, the more options you have. If delayed, tooth loss may be inevitable, and you will have limited options. If you're nervous about care because of bad experiences as a child or horror stories from a family member, sedation may be the way to go for you. Rest assured, you can not only save your smile but make it look and feel as good as it did before, or even better.

SIX

Have No Fear—
Sedation Dentistry Is Here!

It's easy to avoid the dentist due to fear. I experienced it myself as a child. But sweeping it under the rug only makes things worse and unnecessarily expensive, both in terms of cost and life impact. Examples include:

- Inability to enjoy your favorite foods
- Sensitive or uncomfortable teeth
- Lowered self-confidence
- Not participating in family photos
- Losing out on a job promotion or interview
- Dreading social events or staying home
- Poor nutrition
- Gaps between teeth trapping food
- People commenting on your "yellow" teeth

———— • ————

Lean Back and Relax
Can you imagine sitting upright, not reclined, for hours with your dentist's fingers and tools in your mouth? Even minutes

spent like this would be uncomfortable. We did not always have reclining chairs. In 1832, James Snell invented the reclining dental chair. Chairs could fully recline by 1958. Today, chairs have become much more comfortable, even offering massaging and heated backs. Plus, we have overhead technology to allow patients to watch portable devices, to maximize their comfort.

———◆———

If you are fearful, a new and safe oral sedation service may be your answer!

One of my most committed patients suffered from dental anxiety for years. She maintained amazing home care but has a genetic predisposition to gum disease and tooth decay, so she needs to see a dentist more frequently. She tried laughing gas and hated how she felt. General anesthesia was not for her either. One day before preparing her for an implant, we discussed oral sedation. I recommended diazepam (also known as Valium). It's a simple pill taken thirty minutes before treatment. She loved it! She said it was the best experience she'd ever had at the dentist and wondered why she hadn't been given oral sedation years earlier. Now we use it every time she needs a procedure done. No more white knuckles or panic attacks. She's awake, relaxed, and treated safely.

———◆———

It Could Be Worse

In 2009, as a fourth-year dental student, I had a fantastic opportunity to go to Jamaica for a dental mission project. Each day our small group would go into a village about thirty minutes outside of Montego Bay, where eager patients would be lined up out front, waiting for needed dental care. The area had only one public dentist to serve over one hundred thousand people. So when the Jamaica Project from the Virginia Commonwealth University would visit once a year, we students had more than enough work to do.

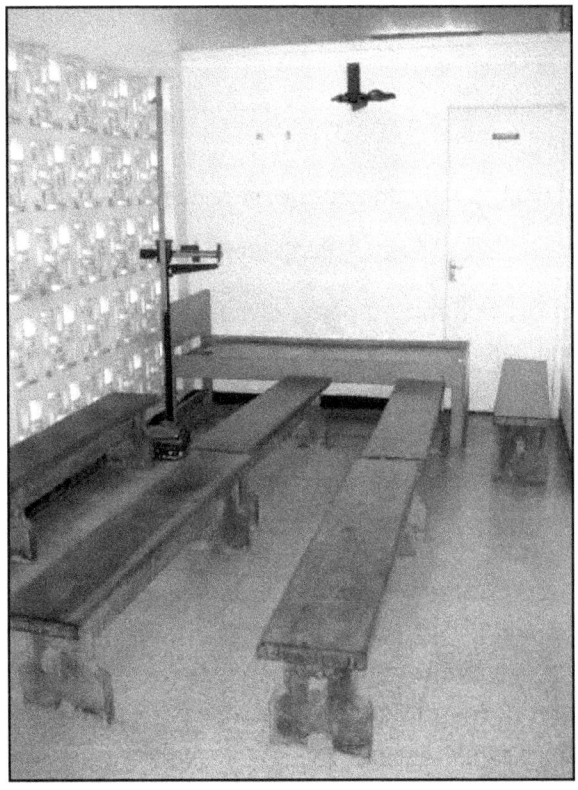

This building served as a church, hospital, and our dental clinic.

The cinder-block building served at each day acted as a medical clinic, dental clinic, and church. There was no modern equipment, so we brought portable instruments and supplies. Here I had my first opportunity to experience upright dentistry. James Snell had a vision of better chair ergonomics and comfort for a reason. It can be difficult to remove some wisdom teeth in perfect conditions, let alone in a humid building with flies, plastic lawn chairs, and built-to-last, tough Jamaican jawbones! Jamaicans are known to have very dense and strong bone, so removing teeth can be challenging, especially with limited resources. But we provided a great service to people in dire need of preventative cleanings, restoring decayed cavities, and removing infected teeth. They had big smiles and were very grateful. One villager even made us a hand-carved Rod of Asclepius (the symbol of healing) in exchange for his dental care. They never complained or took anything we offered for granted. They put their trust in us, and it motivated us to work a full day with very few breaks. It was emotionally overwhelming at first to see the need, but as the days went on, we were able to help many Jamaicans feel better.

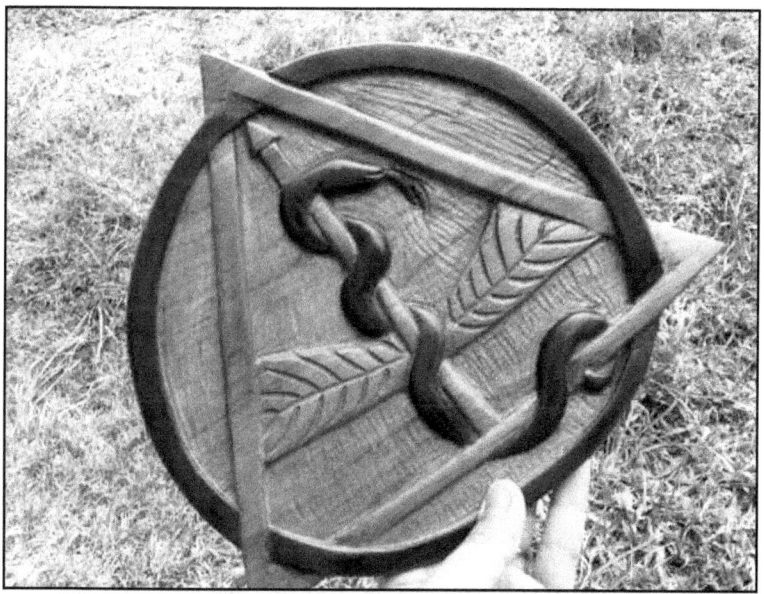

Hand-carved gift from one of the villagers named "Puty."

I'll never forget the pile of medical waste behind the village clinic: used needles and rusty blades and other instruments. Everything was burned each day to remove contaminants. This wasn't the safe red containers to dispose of waste I was used to. We have it good in the United States...really good!

————•◆•————

If you suffer from any dental phobia or if you can't easily sit still in a dentist's chair with your mouth open, sedation dentistry may be the answer for you. Sedation dentistry is a safe and revolutionary service to use when you don't want to hear sounds, experience tastes, or notice smells that will turn your knuckles white. Thanks to modern methods and monitoring equipment, it is easier, safer, and more comfortable than ever.

————•◆•————

Dentists: Pain-Managing Pioneers

2250 BCE *A Babylonian clay tablet is one of the earliest records of chemical pain management for dentistry. Powdered plants were mixed into a cement that was applied to soothe a toothache.*

1723 *Pierre Fauchard, a French dentist, publishes The Surgeon Dentist, A Treatise on Teeth (Le Chirurgien Dentiste). Fauchard is credited as being the "father of modern dentistry" because he was the first to describe a comprehensive practice of dentistry.*

1760 *Issac Greenwood practices as the first US-born dentist.*

1768 *Paul Revere places ads in a Boston newspaper offering his dental services.*

1842 *William Thomas Green Morton, an American dental surgeon, gives the first successful public demonstration of ether anesthesia during surgery.*

1846 *Horace Wells, an American dental surgeon, extracts the first tooth with nitrous oxide.*

1877 Sister Mary Bernard becomes the first nurse anesthetist.

1880s The collapsible metal tube revolutionizes toothpaste and takes it mainstream.

1896 G.V. Black classifies carious lesions—and his classification system is still used today. He publishes the Manual of Operative Dentistry in 1896. (Because I'm a dental nerd, I have collected a couple of his classic operative dentistry textbooks—he was way ahead of his time!)

1904 Novocain is discovered. Although no longer used, it is the precursor for our current local anesthetics.

1953 The American Dental Society of Anesthesiology is founded.

———————•♦•———————

There are multiple levels of sedation used in dentistry, from mild sedation to general anesthesia. Sedation dentistry options vary depending on your needs. The following are examples of differing levels of sedation. As always, discuss these options with a licensed dentist who has advanced training in sedation to find which is best for you.

Mild sedation is commonly used to help people struggling with dental anxiety. This usually comes in the form of inhaling nitrous oxide. It helps you feel relaxed and at ease while you are fully awake. "Laughing gas" treatment is made up primarily of oxygen, so it is safe for most people, it wears off within just a few minutes, and it doesn't impair your ability to drive, think, or work when you are finished with your care. It simply makes you feel "funny" or relaxed and allows the procedure to fly by in your mind. Most often children fall asleep in my chair on nitrous oxide because they are so relaxed. Within five minutes of the completion of your procedure, the laughing gas is 100 percent flushed out of your system, and you are back to being 100 percent you. In my office, this is the most common type of sedation for patient safety and convenience.

Moderate sedation is often called for with procedures where you might need to hold your mouth open for long periods of time or if you are very nervous. This is also not uncommon for patients with special needs, such as those who have involuntary body movements, including bad gag reflexes, or dental anxiety. The sedative agent used in moderate sedation might be a pill or liquid. I've done many of these in my practice, and it works incredibly well. Although I've never had any significant medical problems with this type of sedation, basic monitoring equipment is used to ensure your safety. In my office, we refer to this as our "dental cocktail" to manage anxiety.

The medicine does not directly induce sleep and therefore is a very safe option. While you might fall asleep during the procedure because you are relaxed, you can easily be awakened to answer key questions. Most people smile a lot and feel very happy when they take oral sedatives. Once the procedure is complete, is the sedative is usually allowed to wear off on its own. You should not drive or operate heavy machinery for several hours after being sedated.

Deep sedation puts you at ease during long or invasive procedures such as multiple tooth extractions, multiple teeth restorations and implants, or outpatient oral surgery. Deep sedation is usually administered via a slow-drip IV. It can take a little while for you to get back on your feet after being deeply sedated, so you will need to arrange to have someone drive you and perhaps help you out at home while you're getting back on your feet. Dentists will either administer this on their own or hire a certified dental anesthesiologist.

General anesthesia is a medically induced state of complete unconsciousness. A person under this is unable to feel pain during dental or medical procedures. Usually this is performed in a hospital. General anesthesia combines IV drugs and inhaled gasses and is more than just being asleep—it anesthetizes your brain so that it has zero response to pain signals. A specially trained doctor, dentist, or nurse monitors and manages your body's breathing and other functions while you are unconscious.

———◆———

Dental Sedation has Limited Risks, and the Peaceful Care Is Fantastic!

Anesthesia for dental procedures is generally safe for most adults but does pose some risks. So, make use of it but also make sure you approach it with care.

- *Choose your dentist by researching several. Compare training, testimonials, and number of procedures done.*
- *Talk with your dentist about your medical history. Sleep disorders, weight, and medication are among the things that can complicate sedation.*
- *Be your own advocate. Ask what dose of sedation will be used and if it's within the FDA's recommended levels for your age and health. Review the risks with your dentist. Ask how the dentist monitors vital signs and is prepared for emergencies.*
- *Use the safest and most effective sedation option for your needs. For example, for a single wisdom tooth removal, many of my patients use either oral sedation or nitrous oxide. If you have four impacted wisdom teeth that need removal, you may consider IV or oral sedation for a higher level of relaxation.*

———◆———

SEVEN

Oral Cancer: Striking Us Younger Than Ever Before

I had a friend in high school I will refer to here as JP. JP was diagnosed with oral cancer a few years after we graduated high school. Most of his affected jaw was removed to take out the cancer, and a metal plate replaced it. We lost touch after I moved away for college, but my understanding is after his life-changing surgery, JP was able to raise awareness about oral cancer and spoke with youth organizations and nonprofits to positively influence kids. Unfortunately, he passed away just a few years later, as the aggressive cancer returned. This is one reason annual oral cancer screenings are so important to me: it touched my circle of friends directly. We may have saved JP's life if we had had the technology we do now.

The ADA reports that each year one in ninety-two adults is diagnosed with some form of oral cancer. It commonly appears on the lips, gums, cheeks, tongue, the floor or roof of the mouth, and the throat. Oral cancer occurs when the cells making up your mouth and/or oral cavity mutate. These changes allow cancer cells to continue growing and dividing. The growing number of abnormal cells form an irregular growth. If the tumor or growth is removed quickly (during stage one or stage two of cancer), the outcome is usually very good, with minimal surgery and a speedy recovery.

Oral cancer is an increasing threat to younger people. In 2010, actor Michael Douglas announced that he had oral cancer. He had had a sore throat for a long time and finally went to see a doctor about it. Other warning signs of oral cancer can include redness and irritation, red or white patches, pain, lumps in your mouth, difficulty chewing, and the way your teeth are aligned. Usually a spot that doesn't go away after two weeks needs to be examined and tested. After evaluation and testing, doctors determined Douglas had stage four squamous cell carcinoma oral cancer. He began both radiation and chemotherapy treatments. Despite being diagnosed with such late-stage cancer, he is now cancer-free. Regular checkups monitor his remission. Most people aren't so lucky when they are in stage four—the five-year survival rate is usually less than 50 percent, even after treatment.

The Mayo Clinic lists risk factors as tobacco, heavy alcohol use, and excessive time unprotected in the sun. However, these aren't the primary factors for a rising tide of oral cancer in our country. Until Douglas's very publicized diagnosis, oral cancer was considered a disease of the very old, usually among people who had smoked heavily their whole lives. However, as Douglas said in a 2016 public service announcement for the Oral Cancer Foundation, the fastest growing segment of Americans getting cancers of the mouth are younger people who aren't tobacco users. The human papillomavirus (HPV) is a sexually transmitted virus that can also cause oral cancer. Technically, HPV can even be transferred via saliva. We are now screening for oral cancer at ages thirteen and up on an annual basis and twice a year for high-risk patients.

Prevention

The Mayo Clinic, ADA, and the surgeon general advise stopping use of all tobacco. Smoked or chewed, it exposes your mouth's cells to cancer-causing chemicals. Frequent alcohol exposure also irritates the body's cells, leaving them vulnerable to cancer. I think the public as a whole is much better informed on this than we were even a few decades ago. Most of us understand tobacco is bad, regardless of the form. E-cigarettes and vaping are also hazardous and are showing to be just as harmful as tobacco in many ways.

Eating natural, unprocessed foods not only benefits your oral health but provides antioxidants and vitamins that help strengthen your body's defense systems and skin against cancer.

When you spend time in the sun, wear a wide-brimmed hat and apply lip balm that includes sunscreen. Many of us do these days, especially compared to when my grandparents were kids. Vitamin D is good for our skin, but after fifteen or so minutes of exposure to the sun, sunscreen should be worn. Most of us remember to wear sunblock when we are swimming or at the beach, but what about when we go to the park, run, or play golf?

People who spend a lot of time outdoors have been found to have an increased rate of skin cancer on their lower lips, due to the angle of the sun—men who are less likely to wear lip protection regularly are especially at risk. Many cosmetics contain UV protection, so people who wear makeup are often better protected than those who don't. Fishermen, golfers, bikers, and hikers, be prepared! My wife is a cosmetologist, so recently I asked her to find me an aftershave that contains SPF so I could kill two birds with one stone. My family spends a lot of time hiking, at the lake, or at Grandma's pool, so we keep sunblock and lip balm handy at all times.

How Your Dentist Can Help

Getting checked for oral cancer at the dentist? Yes, it's true. Regular six-month dental checkups include an oral cancer screening (at least once a year in low- to moderate risk patients). If you go to the dentist regularly, your dentist can spot the cancer early. My hygienists and I perform a head and neck exam during each dental checkup. Once a year we use a painless light on our patients for a more in-depth screening. This involves inspecting common areas like the tongue, throat, face, and neck for swelling or abnormal discoloration. If I notice any sign of oral or pharyngeal cancer, we use a cytology test (similar to a pap smear) or remove part of the lesion and send it to an oral pathology lab for review. If it's serious enough, it would be referred to an oral surgeon or head and neck surgeon for surgery.

A few years ago, a friend of one of my hygienists had an abnormal area in the back of his throat that was discovered at his dental checkup during his head and neck exam. They didn't perform biopsies at that office, so he was told he should go see someone who did. He chose not to, because he didn't see the need at the time. He never smoked, drank, or participated in any other high-risk activities in his life. Well, six months later, at his next checkup, there is was, a big cancerous lesion. It almost took his life, and his quality of living was completely disrupted for months because half of his throat had to be removed to get all of the abnormal, cancerous cells out. HPV was identified as the cause. The last I heard, he was doing OK, but he will need to be closely monitored for years to come, and it's a great lesson for us all. You may be vulnerable, even if you don't think you are.

EIGHT

What Kills More People Every Year Than Drunk Drivers? Sleep Apnea

Several years ago, I received a call from a family friend. He was an ex-NFL lineman who had also been a youth football coach to my younger brother for several years. Terry, as I'll call him in this story, had been diagnosed with sleep apnea some time before.

Terry reached out to me because he knew that certain dentists are uniquely able to help with sleep apnea.

Dentists are often the first professionals to notice this problem, and many of us are trained to treat it. Sleep apnea occurs when your muscles relax during sleep, allowing soft tissue to collapse and block your airway. Think of putting a toilet plunger in the toilet bowl and flushing it at the same time. That blocked sensation is similar to what people with sleep apnea suffer (very often unknowingly) during sleep. It is a life-threatening epidemic, and millions of Americans are undiagnosed with it. I see patients with symptoms daily. Fortunately, awareness is starting to gain traction, because more and more patients and outside people are coming to me with questions about it.

Terry was working in California but arranged to stop by my office when he was back home in Utah visiting family. He planned to return in a few weeks to receive his custom oral appliance and start his appliance therapy. Unfortunately, I never saw Terry again. He suffered a massive heart attack that took his life, likely from his sleep condition. I wish I would have known what I know now. I would have reached out to him months earlier to give him an option to sleep better. Prevention saves lives. Poor sleep, especially sleep apnea, has been linked to many diseases, including cancer, diabetes, erectile dysfunction, Alzheimer's, and heart disease. If Terry wasn't being robbed of his oxygen every night from sleep apnea, his heart may have lasted longer. Studies have shown that men over the age of fifty, with a history of high blood pressure and a neck size larger than sixteen inches have a 95 percent chance of suffering with sleep apnea. You can find two great screening tools online. Search "S.T.O.P. B.A.N.G." and the Epworth sleepiness scale. If you score high on either of these, get to a sleep lab or qualified dentist right away for an overnight sleep test and find out why you are having these symptoms. Remember these are screening tools only. While they are usually helpful, I have had patients score low on these tests and yet were still found to have sleep apnea.

Many people don't know the dangers of sleep apnea, but a quick online search will show many stories of people who have died from it—and even unintentionally killed others because of it. Reuters reported in October 2016 on a tour bus driver who crashed into a tractor trailer, killing thirteen and injuring another thirty people. The driver had untreated sleep apnea. In fact, sleep apnea kills more people each year than drunk drivers do. Imagine if you had a sleep disorder and you drove a truck or a school bus for a living. That could be disastrous.

Sleep apnea also leads to other issues, including dry mouth, which can lead to further oral health concerns. There is also a combination of symptoms we know as the bruxism triad, related to sleep apnea. I distinctly remember reading an article in early 2010, just before I graduated dental school. I read it in one of the first online continuing education courses I ever took—and I've been hooked on this science ever since. The research done by Dr. Jeffrey Rouse, a dentist, found a common link among unknowing teeth grinding during sleep, acid reflux (GERD), and sleep apnea. It has been an interesting link for me to study, and I've found countless numbers of my patients in this boat. Often when I see worn teeth on adults, I ask if they have acid reflux and/or heartburn or sleep apnea. Most say yes to at least one. It's also a great screening tool for those who have never received a sleep test to find out if they have any sleep conditions. Since learning of it, I have diagnosed or referred many people with this combination condition.

I asked my friend Scott Schauss, a certificated physician assistant, to share his thoughts on sleep apnea for this book. In his work in sleep medicine, he meets with a lot of patients suffering from sleep apnea. He has a lot of experience in the sleep lab, testing and diagnosing patients with all types of sleep disorders. He and I work together with patients who are diagnosed with mild or moderate obstructive sleep apnea but can't or won't wear a CPAP or similar mask for sleep apnea. So, he refers them to me for oral appliance therapy. Plus, I find so many of my own patients have signs of sleep apnea but have not received a home sleep test, so we get them over to Scott ASAP for a basic or overnight sleep test.

After he shares his expertise, I'll tell you more about treatment options I recommend. With so many sleep-related deaths, effects on our bodies, and links to other medical and dental conditions, I take screening and treating sleep disorders very seriously.

—————◆—————

Destined to Help: Scott Schauss's Story

I always knew that I wanted to work in medicine. I love sports and thought working in sports medicine would be a worthwhile pathway. It didn't quite turn out that way, but looking back, I can say there are no regrets.

It was my second year of physician assistant school, and I was just starting my family medicine clinical rotations with Dr. Seth Wallace. Dr. Wallace also happened to be a board-certified sleep specialist. Naturally, during my time with Dr. Wallace, I was exposed to sleep medicine. Over time I came to enjoy it, I found my interests changing, and after graduation, I began my career in sleep medicine.

What attracts me the most to sleep medicine is how much of a positive impact I can have on someone's health. Most of my patients who are suffering from a sleep disorder(s) have very poor qualities of life, not only on a day-to-day basis but long-term as well. As supposed to treating hypertension for example, treating sleep disorders is very gratifying because of the immediate and recognizable impact it has.

OSA: The Most Common Sleep Apnea

Most of my patients suffer from a sleep disorder called obstructive sleep apnea, or OSA. OSA is when your oxygen levels are lowered in the bloodstream due to the airway closing off. Simply put, you are suffocating. OSA is the most common sleep disorder and impacts roughly 25 million Americans. To give you some perspective, roughly 43.3 million Americans suffer from high blood pressure or hypertension.

We need oxygen to survive, and without it our bodies begin to shut down. To give you an understanding of how serious this can be, the worst I have seen in a patient was breathing disturbances occurring 160 times each hour. That is 2.66 events per minute that are lasting at least 10 seconds each and dropping the oxygen 3 percent or more from baseline. While it is true that our bodies are designed to keep us alive in such moments, the day-to-day and even long-term ramifications can be quite severe and debilitating.

Who Is Most at Risk for OSA?

Notable risk factors for OSA include advancing age, being male, and obesity. In fact, obesity is probably the strongest risk factor, with 80 percent of anyone with a body mass index of 40 having OSA. Other factors include family history, neck size, and how closed off the back of your throat or airway is.

OSA Symptoms

The big three signs of OSA include loud and excessive snoring and pauses in breathing, followed by a gasp for air. Symptoms are generally going to be complaints of unrefreshing sleep with difficulty getting out of bed in the morning, memory loss, mood shifts, and daytime fatigue with excessive daytime sleepiness being a major complaint. The reason why daytime sleepiness is a predominating symptom is that at night, every time you have a breathing disturbance, your body wakes you up, so you breathe again. This is how you survive. It also means you never get a full night's rest.

As you can imagine or have even experienced yourself, it is very difficult to have an optimal quality of life when you are constantly sleepy and/or fatigued. Most people with OSA suffer in all aspects of their lives; school, work, relationships, even personal health. The estimated economic cost of undiagnosed OSA was nearly $150 billion in 2015.

Dangers of Living with OSA

This leads me to discuss some of the dangers of OSA. One of the most common things that I see in my clinic is drowsy driving. Some patients have been fortunate enough to have never fallen asleep at the wheel, but others have. Imagine if your family members were involved in a major accident due to a drowsy driver. Paints a realistic picture, doesn't it? Please never drive drowsy.

In addition to drowsy driving, most patients will run the risk of developing or worsening existing medical conditions. In fact, those with sleep apnea have a two to three times more risk for developing atrial fibrillation, an erratic and *dangerous heart rhythm that may contribute to other dangerous health risks. Other risks include heart attacks, strokes, developing or worsening diabetes or hypertension, Alzheimer's, dementia, and Parkinson's. Quite frankly, there isn't an area of the body that OSA does not impact.*

OSA Solutions

Hopefully you're not discouraged at this point. There are ways to lower your risk. The first step is to see and consult a sleep specialist for further diagnosis. Diagnosis is done through a sleep study, either at home or in the lab. That decision is made on factors such as your comorbidities or existing health issues, risk factors, insurance, and standard of practices. Once testing is completed, the best way to treat sleep apnea is with a continuous positive airway machine otherwise known as CPAP. Other forms of therapy include mandible advancement devices, oral surgery and/or nerve stimulators. For example, in mild, straightforward OSA cases, a mandibular advancement device can be very effective and appropriate. In all cases, please consult with your sleep specialist before therapy is started.

As important as CPAP or other treatment modalities are, weight loss is crucial. I'm asked every day on how to get rid of OSA all together. The answer in 95 to 99 percent of cases is, simply, lose enough weight and there is a good chance that your OSA will decrease in severity or go away all together. Obstructive sleep apnea is a serious disease and at times life threatening, but with the proper diagnosis and management, it can be controlled and lower the risk of negative outcomes.

———•◆•———

Is A CPAP The Best Option?

Scott shared a lot of great information. Now I'm going to bring us back to my friend Terry, with whom I introduced this chapter. He didn't reach out to me to diagnose his sleep apnea—that part was already done. He reached out to me to help him better treat it, so he could breathe while he slept. He'd been prescribed a CPAP machine but wasn't wearing it because it wasn't comfortable for him. He knew I offered an alternative solution that was much more comfortable.

CPAP, which stands for Continuous Positive Airway Pressure, is the most common treatment for sleep apnea. A CPAP machine is made up of a house and full-face mask or nosepiece to keep oxygen moving steadily into a patient. But CPAP can be, to put it bluntly, a real pain in the mouth to deal with. To some, a CPAP is like Darth Vader's mask. It can even make some patients feel claustrophobic. In addition, it can take a few tries to get the mask to fit properly. The face is a unique surface; this is definitely no "one size fits all" machine. Any problems with the machine's fit can lead to the mask rubbing the skin, can lead to dry mouth, and can lead to the patient even removing the CPAP in their sleep.

Oral appliance therapy that dentists provide is an increasingly preferred form of treatment for OSA. This is due to the high rejection rate (up to 50 percent) of CPAP therapy and the fact that oral appliances are much more convenient, portable, and easy to care for. Oral appliance therapy uses a mouthguard-like device to maintain an open, unobstructed airway while you sleep. They are typically as simple to wear as most retainers. Even though it feels like a hockey puck in your mouth when you first receive it, an oral appliance wins hands down next to a CPAP in the comfort department. For most people, the jaw and muscles get used to it usually after a few days or weeks. Studies show appliances work for over 80 percent of people. I have gone through the process myself, from a home sleep test to having an appliance made. I haven't been diagnosed with sleep apnea, but since I discuss it with so many patients so often, I wanted to gain a better understanding of the process. I am picky about my mouth, and I slept a full night, well rested on my first try with my dual-arch (upper and lower mouthpiece) sleep appliance.

There are two ways in which oral appliance therapy works to open your airway:

- By repositioning your lower jaw, it keeps your throat muscles lightly engaged as you sleep, preventing them from collapsing.
- Oral appliances can also move your tongue forward, keeping it from falling back and blocking the throat.

Conclusion

One in five adults has OSA, but most of those people go undiagnosed, suffering without realizing it until the condition causes a major health concern. Just as sleep apnea can cause problems throughout your body, if you treat the rest of your body well, you can counteract that sleep condition. Weight loss is an incredible natural cure for sleep apnea, but I have seen many patients at a healthy weight who have a small airway or a large tongue and tonsils or who are at a high risk from medical conditions or lifestyle habits and who need sleep apnea therapy. Keep in mind that CPAP therapy is a great option and is still the first line of defense for severe OSA or for those with central sleep apnea (CSA, a neurological type of sleep apnea). Dentists have techniques to help those with OSA comfortably and simply manage their apnea without adding a cumbersome machine to their bedtime routine.

Even those who are not candidates for an oral appliance should be aware of acid and heartburn issues or teeth that are chipping or wearing prematurely. Nighttime grinding for just one night's sleep has been equated to as much force as up to ten days of chewing. So, uncontrolled teeth grinding will wear your teeth out ten times faster. Many sleep apnea patients also require a medication for acid reflux and may need to wear a bite splint with their CPAP to protect from the devastating effects of nighttime grinding. Most of those who do wear a CPAP should also wear a bite guard or occlusal splint to protect from the damage of grinding. Ask your dentist if you have signs of accelerated wear.

If you suspect someone has sleep apnea or notice your partner gasping in bed or sleeping restlessly, set up a sleep test with a qualified sleep lab today or get to a dentist trained in sleep apnea therapy for a treatment plan and referral. You could greatly reduce avoidable medical costs, improve quality of living, or even save your life, or the life of someone you care about.

NINE

Dental Implants: The Best Natural Tooth Replacement

Uncontrolled decay and/or periodontal disease leads to tooth loss. No matter how much we try to prevent certain oral health issues, the simple fact is sometimes life happens. Usually we can save teeth, but when some are so far gone, it typically isn't worth the time or investment to save a tooth or multiple teeth. Today, we are living longer, and tooth decay and gum disease are becoming more and more common for certain groups, and we have more access to processed foods than ever before. Plus, there are genetic, medical, and lifestyle factors to consider. So, it's likely you will lose a tooth due to decay, gum disease, or accident at some point in your life. The good news is technology for replacing missing teeth, should you ever need it, is more natural and better than ever.

The old phrase "long in the tooth" is true as we keep our teeth longer. But when they get too "long" they should be removed. When gum disease gets very severe, our bodies will naturally start to reject the teeth, seeing them as a "splinter" that is no longer part of the core system to keep us healthy and protected. It's part of our natural defense system. I use the five-year rule: if a restored tooth will likely last five years or more, I will go to great lengths to save it; if it won't, I consider a replacement option such as dental implants.

Remember when I mentioned my wife's baby tooth "blowing up" on her during pregnancy? Well, not long after our son arrived, Megan received a dental implant to replace the now empty space. Within four months, she had a porcelain tooth over a titanium root, which she could floss and eat with: a dental implant. No one could tell the difference between that tooth and her other ones, and our friends are still surprised when they find out she has an artificial tooth because it blends in so well. (Thankfully, she likes her dentist too!) Even when you're carefully diligent with your home care, you may still find yourself with a gap in your pearly whites someday. A friend of mine lost his two front teeth before he was twenty-one years old, playing racquetball... *whack!* His Christmas wish that year was just his two front teeth.

Thanks to modern methods, he got them back!

Dental technology has advanced well beyond your grandmother's partial bridges and dentures. Dental implants are replacement, artificial tooth roots. Unlike dentures, they look, feel, and function like your natural teeth. You can floss between them and eat the foods you love, and no one but you and your dentist know that they aren't the natural teeth God gave you. Dental implants help preserve your jawbone's structure, as well as your facial structure, so you don't end up looking like Popeye the Sailorman. Implants act like teeth to our bone cells, which stimulates the jawbone, helping it maintain its density. This keeps you looking young because your cheeks do not start to collapse, therefore reducing the chance of extra wrinkles and skin folds from an overclosed bite.

Missing Teeth—Does It Really Matter?

You may be tempted to try to live with the gap left by a missing tooth. It is "just one tooth," after all. But the loss of a tooth can affect your mouth in multiple ways. At first, it can impair your ability to chew food and perhaps give you an unappealing smile. In time, the structural loss of the tooth usually causes the surrounding teeth to twist and migrate toward the empty space. (You can watch a short video simulation on implants on the bonus website when you register your copy of this book.) This greatly increases your chances of suffering chips and fractures in the remaining teeth and gum disease due to poor bone levels and attachment loss of tooth ligaments.

Placing Dental Implants

The process starts with your dentist examining the area and taking a few X-rays. It's important to make sure you have sufficient bone structure to place a dental implant root. If there is not enough bone structure to support an implant, you might need to have a bone graft, sinus lift, or ridge expansion. It sounds more complicated than it is. For most people, this can be done in under an hour, and your dentist will use a local anesthetic to make your mouth numb and comfortable. Afterward, you usually need to eat soft foods for a few days, but otherwise you don't have to miss much time from work or school (unless you really want to!).

The main drawback to bone grafting or ridge expanding if done at a separate time from the tooth removal is added cost and time, and it may add three to nine months before your missing tooth is restored. It is usually worth it to have a bone replacement socket graft at the time of removal. You will heal quicker and more comfortably, and it prevents your jaw from shrinking or changing shape. Think of it like removing a dead tree from your yard. You are better off putting top soil and fertilizer in the empty hole where the tree roots were, than just leaving an opening there and watering it. Earth may shift around that hole in ways you don't want it to. A bone replacement graft preserves the site until you are ready to get a new tooth. Now we can even place the new root at the same time as removing the dead or damaged one, which means expedited healing and reduced cost and time to completion. Plus, you are already numb, so no extra dental visits!

Mini Size, Maximum Benefit

Mini dental implants are similar to regular dental implants, just narrower. These implants are beneficial when your underlying bone has been compromised by gum disease or other dental issues or you have been missing teeth for many years and aren't a good candidate for ridge grafting (bone replacement). In most cases where the bone is very narrow or has been missing a tooth for many years, it is likely able to support a mini dental implant. Placing mini implants in the mouth can take as little as one appointment. We can use sedation or local anesthesia alone, and generally you don't need stitches or have much bleeding, if any at all. It amazes people every day!

To place a dental implant, I make a tiny opening in your jawbone (or use the one that's already there if we are taking out the tooth at the same time). The opening is less than 1.5 mm, or about the width of a lead pencil tip. Then, I gently twist a titanium implant into place that is slightly wider than the hole. This way, we usually have little or no bleeding, because the wider implant "corks" up the hole for quick healing and integration. With such a small opening, there is very little surgery involved in many cases.

Once the implant has fully integrated into your jaw (usually two to four months for a single tooth implant, less time for some multiple implant cases), we move on to restoring it. This requires taking a silicone impression, which will serve as a guide for our off-site dental lab technician to mill or fabricate a custom porcelain or ceramic tooth for you. We pour a stone model or create a digital model from a scan and design the abutment (post that attaches to the implant) and crown, bridge, or snap-in bridge (the covering over the abutment that allows you to chew and looks and feels just like a real tooth). Once your restoration is ready, we will call you back in to attach an abutment and place the restoration that you will smile and chew with. Think of the implant root like the basement in your home, the abutment like the main level of your house, and the restoration like the roof. The three work in tandem, tightly and comfortably, usually without any numbing or anesthetic in the final stage(s).

Today we have many restorative options, which allow for a wide range of costs for care, ranging from basic to advanced options. When you buy a car, you can get a standard model, mid-range model, or the high-end version. There are clear differences among the three, but all of these treatment options have their place depending on the patients wants and needs. Today, all of the options are light-years ahead of the dentures of old that often fit like "socks on a rooster." Our jawbones shrink every year the longer we are without teeth, so dentures fit looser and looser over time. Implants, on the other hand, make the body and jawbone believe real teeth are still in the jaw, which prevents bone from rapidly shrinking, as it does with tooth loss.

———— ♦ ————

Cock-A-Doodle-Tooth!

It may not be too surprising that people have been developing basic toothbrushes and toothpastes for thousands of years, but I think it's fascinating that people have been experimenting and succeeding with dental implants for a very long time too.

We have proof of replacement teeth, carved from oxen bones, as early as 500 BCE. Radiographs of Mayan mandibles dating from 600 CE show bone formation around stone implants. Scientists have found four-thousand-year-old Chinese implants carved of bamboo pegs. A 2,300-year-old iron tooth was recently found among real teeth in a Celtic grave in France. Researchers believe they were placed to improve the smile after death and probably didn't have it hammered into place while alive. Thank goodness! There's also a skull dating to ancient America containing a "tooth" made of sea coral. It was probably tapped into place while the person was alive. Since coral is naturally coated with hydroxyapatite, which our body loves, it integrated well throughout the rest of the person's life!

In the 1700s, Dr. John Hunter was experimenting in dentistry. He implanted an underdeveloped tooth into the comb of a rooster. The rooster's blood vessels grew into the tooth, securing the tooth in the comb. But the real father of modern dental implants is the Swedish orthopedic surgeon Dr. Per-Ingvar Brånemark, though he landed in that role rather accidentally. In 1952, he and his research team were studying the body's healing process. One of their experiments involved implanting optical devices in rabbits' legs, so they could monitor what was happening. Those devices happened to be in titanium cases. When Brånemark tried to remove the devices, he found that the metal had fused to the bone.

Brånemark coined the term for this technique that we still use today, "Osseointegration", and he further concluded that titanium could be used to anchor teeth to the jawbone. The New York Times reported further that Brånemark's first dental implant patient was treated in the mid-1960s. The patient had not only no lower teeth but also a cleft palate and jaw deformities. The procedure gave the man four dental implants that allowed him to eat, chew, and smile until his death—four decades later.

We have studies going back thirty and even forty years on implants. They work very well, with a 90–97 percent success rate. I have found that to be true with my own patients—we have better success with implants than with many root canals! They are becoming the standard of care for missing teeth, as dentures and partials usually require changing neighboring teeth, decrease home hygiene ability, and cover or change our ability to taste as well. Some of my implant patients forget which tooth is the replacement, because they look and feel so natural.

Care of Dental Implants

Once your implants are placed in your mouth, you need to care for them like you would care for your natural teeth, in some cases more. This means you need to brush and floss them as well as rinse your mouth regularly. In addition, it's vital to visit your dentist every six months for your professional dental cleaning and exam appointments. If you follow these steps and those we discussed previously, these implants can last for many years, even a lifetime.

TEN

How to Choose
the Right Dentist for You

Here are a few suggestions on how to choose the right dentist for you:

How to Find a Dentist

- Find an office that focuses on relationships and customer service. Dentistry is more about people than it is teeth.
- Read online reviews. Be fair in your study of the reviews— we are all human, and some people who leave comments have unrealistic expectations, and some reviews may be fabricated for good or bad. Someone with a solid online presence is usually someone who takes a lot of pride in the care for their patients.
- Ask your family, friends, neighbors, and coworkers for recommendations.
- Don't base your decision primarily on price. Price is a valid consideration for most of us, but you'll actually save more money and better preserve your health by finding the right match. If you change offices too often, you will likely experience inconsistencies in your care or conflicting information. Getting a treatment plan you feel comfortable with and sticking to it

is your best option. (Note: Today, some of the big box dental chains have "quotas" on how many root canals or crowns they want to place in a day—don't become a number! Most dentists have good intentions, but watch out for certain offices that push treatment on you.)

- Contact your state dental society. These societies can also help you find low-cost clinics or dental schools in your area if you are unemployed or have financial hardship.
- Ask your physician.
- Don't go primarily for insurance. Most dental plans allow you to see any dentist you choose, even if they aren't on "the list." With medical costs rising, fewer implant and preventative dental services are covered by many plans, so doing what's right for you matters more than what your plan dictates. In my office, we are very insurance-friendly and work with most plans. However, we don't let the plan dictate; we let the patient choose what's best for them. There are great offices out there offering the same level of care. Find one that suits you.
- Find an office with convenient times that work with your schedule. Extra time off work may cost you more in time and salary than it would by trying to save a few bucks.
- If you are uninsured for dentistry, like 40 percent of Americans are, find an office that accepts payment plans or offers an insurance-alternative membership plan. You don't need insurance to see the dentist any more than you need health insurance to exercise. Home care is priority number one for your oral health; a dental office you know and trust is a close number two.
- Ask what preventative services are offered. Does the office offer digital technology? Oral cancer screenings? Periodontal mapping? Adult fluoride varnish? Home care kits? Dry mouth programs? Helpful home handouts and videos? Before and after success stories?

How to Choose a Dentist from the Narrowed-Down List

Finding a new dentist is about more than just making an appointment with the first name your coworker suggests or with the first clinic you see on a billboard. If you are uncertain, call or visit a few offices. When you visit, ask them questions and ask yourself questions about how you feel when you're there. Trust is key to any relationship, and that's what you need to have the best outcome: a long-term relationship. I know firsthand that the phones get busy, but your dentist should be willing to set up a time to talk in person, face-to-face. In my office, we set aside time for a personal interview of each new patient before we begin any care. Sometimes a patient isn't the right fit for us, and we can make a referral to someone who is and who will care for their needs. A proper interview and introduction ensures our patients are aware of costs, expectations, and treatment options ahead of time. Be informed before someone performs. Here are a few other things to think about:

- Does the staff seem happy on the phone and in person? Do they seem to love helping people like you?
- Are the office hours convenient for your schedule? How are emergencies handled outside of office hours?
- Is the clinic easy for you to get to?
- Do they have a digital intraoral camera? It's a painless way for you to see what your providers see, but on a big screen.
- What is the dentist's approach to preventive dentistry?
- If you or your family experiences dental anxiety, then what type of anesthesia is the dentist certified to administer?
- What are the differences between using insurance and paying out of pocket? Often there is a prepayment savings if you pay for your services by cash or check in full. Some offices now offer plans for patients without insurance—a growing need.
- Are payment plans available if you need major work done?

- What areas of dentistry do the dentists in this practice love to do? What is their passion in helping patients?
- Does the whole office, from waiting room to treatment room, appear clean and orderly?
- And, most importantly, ask the dentist: Why should I have my care and/or work done here?

Considering Special Needs

If you have special health considerations, related to your mouth or other parts of your body, talk to prospective dentists about those needs too before you make your first appointment. You have read this book. You are informed. You deserve high-quality care, and the kind of care that works best will be different for everyone.

Questions you might ask include:

- What training or experience in working with patients with my condition(s) does the office have?
- Do they take the time to understand my needs and my desired outcome(s)?
- Is the office physically accessible to me?
- Do I "feel" the dentist cares about building a long-term relationship to care for me? (Not just drill-fill-bill…)

ELEVEN

The Straight Truth About a Crooked Smile

Straightening for Kids and Teens

Nowadays you'll see teens and older children smiling with colorful elastics and metal or porcelain braces on their teeth everywhere you go. Braces have been shown to help developing adolescents improve the alignment of their teeth, expand narrow jaws to a fuller, more natural shape, and even reduce sleep apnea risks, thanks to widening the airway. We are often treating at an earlier age, which gives more options, requires less overall treatment time, and offers a better outcome.

Some children and teens should have surgery, a retainer, or an expander during or prior to their first stage of orthodontic treatment. Expanders work incredibly well and are also believed to prevent or reduce sleep apnea if applied during the years while our bones are still developing. Many baby boomers had teeth extracted as part of their orthodontic treatment or due to crowding. This is much less common now. I've removed crowded teeth on a select few of my patients, and it's only been a single tooth instead of the old way of two to four teeth removed. Some still need removal for oversized or undersized jaws, but most patients don't, thanks to newer orthodontic technology. Plus, we see a higher rate of sleep apnea in patients who had extra teeth removed, because removing needed teeth can shrink the jaws and mouth, effectively narrowing the airway. If your child has sleeping issues and/or an overbite or crooked teeth, get them in to a qualified dentist or orthodontist by age seven for an evaluation. They may not need treatment, but you can map out a plan that can really save time and drastically improve the outcome.

Straightening for Adults

Straightening isn't just for kids anymore. More and more adults are realizing the health and confidence benefits of a revitalized smile. I've even done tooth straightening on patients in their seventies. I had braces myself for the first time back in 2012, thanks to the fine work by a good friend of mine. It was a great experience for me, and I can really relate to my own patients now. I never had braces (or "train tracks" as some call them...) as a teenager, but I had an overlapped crossbite on a few of my back teeth and a few gaps and crowding that I didn't like in the front. Many of my family and friends remarked, "You have nice teeth," or, "Why do you need braces?" Did I absolutely need them? No. But like many lifestyle improvements, I've never looked back. I'd do it all over again if I had to. My wife and I still look at before and after photos and are amazed. If you would like to learn more about your teeth straightening options, and to see before and after photos or real cases, please visit my website.

I'm a big wimp, so I thought I'd be sore or annoyed by having all that hardware in my mouth. Truthfully, I remember my lips feeling chafed and rubbed for about the first week of my treatment. I used lots of ortho wax on the brackets. After that first week, I took Tylenol or over-the-counter pain medication for a day or two after each of my monthly visits. I didn't have any soreness I couldn't manage, and I didn't use wax for the remainder of my care. If I can do it, you can too.

Today, you have many options to improve the health and appearance of your smile: metal braces, clear braces, clear retainers (such as Invisalign or Clear Correct), and even short-term braces. These treatments can dramatically improve the way your bite feels, the ability for you to clean between teeth that have gaps or are overlapped or have very tight spots, and even the brightness of your smile. Plus, your confidence may hit an all-time high. I've had multiple patients who were graduating or getting married, and we were able to successfully hit the deadlines for their big days, which wasn't an option in years past. Years ago, thick crowns/veneers or metal braces were the only two good options and were at quite different ends of the spectrum. Today, we offer many combinations to find the recipe that's right for you.

Solid Reasons to Beautify That Smile and How We Do It

According to the ADA, there are many reasons to have an abnormal bite or misaligned teeth corrected with straightening. These include:

- Increased risk for tooth decay due to inability to clean or floss optimally
- Higher chance of periodontal disease or gingivitis
- Loss of teeth from wear or misalignment
- Affected speech and/or chewing
- Abnormal wearing away of enamel
- Jaw or TMJ problems
- Sleep apnea or breathing issues

In my office, we treat many adults for misaligned teeth. The most common way I help adults is with short-term orthodontics, or STO, which usually involves a six-to-nine-month treatment plan. About 80 percent of my adult patients choose this option for straightening. People love it because the braces are white or clear, it doesn't require as much treatment time as conventional braces, and they get results fast. We focus on the teeth you see when you smile, which allows us to give you a new smile in months instead of years. Usually we can transform a smile between one six-month checkup to the next. Plus, we also incorporate implants for missing teeth and/or resin bonding to correct chipped, worn, or misshapen teeth for our best outcomes. What's really great is we can now design digital models and workflows from a scan of your teeth. This 3-D treatment plan allows you to preview the expected progress and outcome of your teeth, even before you start. Plus, it makes our movements of teeth incredibly accurate. These are a lot of fun because not only do we see our patients' health improve but their whole demeanor changes and confidence goes through the roof.

For those who need more advanced correction with their bite or jaw, I use a system such as Invisalign to straighten and align their smiles, which is generally an eighteen-to-twenty-four-month treatment time. For many children and those with very complex orthodontic needs, I refer them to an orthodontist. I studied different orthodontic systems while training in dental school, and I also took the Invisalign training course. I was very interested (and still am) in comprehensive dentistry. One of the things I love most is when we get to integrate multiple disciplines of dentistry, such as bonding and straightening to make over a smile. After dental school, I have spent countless hours studying and being involved in continuing education courses on implants, orthodontics, and restorative dentistry. It's a lot of fun to put these techniques or services to work simultaneously, and my patients love it!

———— ◆ ————

Living in the Shadows

There's an area at the corners of our smile we refer to as the buccal corridor. It is the space between your upper back teeth and your lips and cheeks. This area may look dark, yellow, or gray when we have gapped, crooked, or overlapped teeth. Many people have tried home whitening strips and don't feel they get much improvement. That's because the spaces and dark areas show through the teeth. While living in the shadows, our whitened enamel doesn't show nearly as well as it could. When teeth are rotated or moved into a better position, we naturally see more white enamel, even without veneers. But couple whitening and veneers with a newly straightened smile, and you'll have the brightest smile you've ever seen.

———— ◆ ————

Straight teeth go way beyond improved appearance. Our mouths feel better, and we can clean them so much easier when they are lined up in an ideal position. Remember when I wrote about periodontal health as the number one reason for tooth loss in adults? A properly aligned smile can improve and even prevent this disease. Plus, we can chew, eat, and speak better with a well-rounded smile. I've treated countless diseased teeth where the one across from it doesn't touch or there are gaps. You know what commonly happens? You guessed it: gum disease and/or decay. As we chew, our teeth naturally touch each other to grind our food, which also helps clean our teeth (especially with coarse, natural foods). When they don't touch or when we have gaps, food collects and sits there longer than it should, even when we brush and floss. When teeth and jaws are in their proper places, we instantly drop our risk of future decay and gingivitis.

Think of your car or bike: as long as the wheels are out of alignment, it doesn't matter how good the rubber tires are—they'll wear out faster and you'll have a rougher ride. Our teeth and bite are very similar: the better they line up, the longer our teeth last and the easier they are to clean.

Retainers

Yes, you'll need them if you straighten. Retainers are the best solution to secure all the hard work you've gone through. I've met with countless adults who had braces during childhood, or even twice in their lives, and still they suffer from relapse—teeth shifting back to being crooked. Most of the time, the relapse is due to losing or not wearing their retainers. Think of it like getting in shape. Once you cut out the sweets, add exercise, and get into a great routine, that doesn't mean your body will stay that way on its own. It's your responsibility to keep it there. There are few things in our bodies that do not require upkeep for the best result. Even those who've never had braces or are happy with their teeth will likely experience some shifting during their lifetime, possibly due to wisdom teeth, decay, gum disease, or tooth loss. Retention for your new smile is the most important part of your treatment—it's up to you!

For each of my orthodontic patients, I make both a fixed (bonded wire) and removable (clear tray) retainer once they complete their treatment. This way they have double coverage to protect the integrity of their new smile. Removable retainers should be worn daily, for as little as fifteen minutes, or overnight, depending on your dentist's or orthodontist's recommendation. I've found it's more about the consistency than the duration. Our mouths need a "little reminder" every day to stay put. Plus, you have the option to use whitening gel in your clear retainer. Fixed retainers should stay bonded for life, usually behind four to six of your top front and/or bottom front teeth only. They are concealed so no one sees them, and we give out special toothpicks and floss to clean around them, so you don't get extra plaque buildup. I have both a top and bottom bonded wire in my own mouth, and I have forgotten about them, and no one else even knows they are there.

Conclusion

Whether short-term or conventional orthodontics is right for you, the great news is that you have options. By following a plan, having your braces or trays adjusted regularly, and most importantly, by retaining them, you'll have a long-lasting smile that will stay healthier and brighter.

TWELVE

Change Begins Today

I hope you enjoyed reading this book as much as I enjoyed writing it. I am passionate about dentistry—just ask my wife; it's one thing I can talk about for hours. She always knows when she walks into a room and teeth have been the topic of discussion—I light up. Sharing knowledge is how we can grow quicker and more successfully as a community and society. It's a great opportunity to learn from others so we can experience the benefits of new dentistry. That's what prevention is all about.

As I mentioned, my goal is to get the whole country to a dentist at least once per year. It will start with my local community, then the city, state, region, and finally, the whole country. This is a huge goal, and I don't have nearly enough resources, yet! Together we'll get there—this book is my start. As people gain awareness and the value of oral health is better understood, progress will happen, lives will be improved, and people will feel better about going to the dentist, knowing what to do at home, and instilling best practices in their own families.

If you have questions or would like more information on improving your oral health, you may reach me at the contact information contained within this book. If you know someone who has questions, is nervous, or doesn't like the dentist, share this book with them. They might learn a few things that can make their life better and healthier. As we continue to evolve dental technology, access to care, our lifestyles, and our diets, our community will be enriched. Join me in the movement for preventative dentistry and total-body health that starts with the gateway to the body: the mouth. Finally, remember the words of Mother Teresa: "We shall never know all the good that a simple smile can do." Start today by sharing your smile with someone else.

Resources

The following provides direction to further detail on some of the information provided in this book. Please contact my office if you have any questions.

Preface

To unlock special extras and free bonus content mentioned in this book, visit pinecrestdds.com/book-extras.

For more information on the CDC's findings about dentist visits, please see https://www.cdc.gov/nchs/fastats/dental.htm.

Information about reasons why adults do not seek dental care, as found in a study by the Health Policy Institute of the American Dental Association (ADA), is at *Why Adults Forgo Dental Care: Evidence from a New National Survey* (2014), https://www.ada.org/~/media/ADA/Science%20and%20Research/HPI/Files/HPIBrief_1114_1.ashx.

Chapter 1

For extra knowledge on gum disease, tooth decay, and home health, including before and after photos of straightened smiles, visit www.pinecrestdds.com/book-extras.

Information on the National Institute of Dental and Craniofacial

Research's findings about cavities can be found at https://www.nidcr.nih.gov/DataStatistics/FindDataByTopic/DentalCaries/DentalCariesAdults20to64.htm.

The National Institute of Dental and Craniofacial Research, a part of the National Institutes of Health, has found that 26 percent of adults ages twenty to sixty-four have untreated tooth decay: https://www.nidcr.nih.gov/DataStatistics/FindDataByTopic/DentalCaries/DentalCariesAdults20to64.htm.

If you'd like to read more about twelve-year-old Deamonte Driver and how tooth decay can lead to loss of life, search online for his name. He died in 2007 in Maryland.

A Pew Charitable Trust study offers more information on the high cost of untreated dental issues: http://www.pewtrusts.org/en/research-and-analysis/analysis/2015/06/19/millions-of-medicaid-dollars-spent-on-dental-emergencies.

The number of emergency room visits due to toothaches is rising; here is one source for information on that: https://www.cbsnews.com/news/more-americans-visit-er-for-costly-and-inefficient-dental-care/.

Grand Rapids, Michigan, was the first city to add sodium fluoride to public water systems: https://www.ada.org/en/publications/ada-news/2015-archive/september/ada-hosts-celebration-of-70-years-of-water-fluoridation.

President Harry S. Truman established the National Institute of Dental Research and initiating federal funding for dental research: https://www.nidcr.nih.gov/research/ResearchResults/NewsReleases/ArchivedNewsReleases/NewsReleases2008/NIDCRTurns60.htm.

The most common reason for World War II draft rejection was the would-be soldier having too few teeth because he had experienced dental decay: https://report.nih.gov/NIHfactsheets/ViewFactSheet.aspx?csid=129.

Further information on sealants may be found at http://onlinelibrary.wiley.com/doi/10.1111/j.1834-7819.1997.tb00127.x/pdf.

Information on fluoride varnish may be found at https://www.science-daily.com/releases/2000/04/000413145117.htm.

See the differences among restorative, onlay, and crown options at https://dentagama.com/news/what-is-the-difference-between-inlay-onlay-overlay-and-pinlay.

If you'd like more information on Harvard University's study on periodontal disease and pancreatic cancer, look to this press release: http://archive.sph.harvard.edu/press-releases/2007-releases/press01162007b.html.

More information on the Royal College of Surgeons work on gum health and blood cloths is at https://www.ncbi.nlm.nih.gov/pmc/articles/PMC5574023/.

You can learn more about Perio Protect at https://www.perioprotect.com/.

Chapter 2

To obtain a free copy of my personal home health routine, and some valuable bonus oral health content, please visit pinecrestdds.com/book-extras.

Learn more about what people notice first (hint: your smile) when they meet you: http://1001dentaltips.com/2017/03/14/what-people-notice-first-when-they-meet-someone.

More information about the CDC's ruling on chronic disease and oral health is at https://www.cdc.gov/healthywater/hygiene/disease/dental_caries.html.

Is a loved one begging for a new car? Remind them of this MIT study about the power of the toothbrush: http://news.mit.edu/2003/lemelson.

To learn about this history of toothbrushes, including how important Americans consider them, see this article by another dentist in the *Huffington Post* (it's part of a series!): https://www.huffingtonpost.com/thomas-p-connelly-dds/mouth-health-how-long-hav_b_683535.html.

Information on the CDC fluoride studies can be found at https://www.cdc.gov/fluoridation/statistics/cost.htm.

Here is one study on the erosive properties of sports drinks, from 2012: http://onlinelibrary.wiley.com/doi/10.1111/j.1834-7819.2012.01708.x/pdf.

To see photos of my wisdom teeth experiment, visit pinecrestdds.com/drink-damage.

If you want to learn more or request some free xylitol candy samples, visit pinecrestdds.com/xylitol.

Chapter 3

For more information on total health, visit: www.pinecrestdds.com/book-extras.

For more on the documentary I mentioned, visit: sayahhthemovie.com.

Regarding the *Journal of Periodontology* and the *American Journal of Cardiology* review of data on the links between periodontology and heart health, see https://www.webmd.com/oral-health/features/healthy-teeth-healthy-heart.

To learn more about pregnancy and oral health, visit https://www.colgate.com/en-us/oral-health/life-stages/oral-care-during-pregnancy/pregnancy-prenatal-care-and-oral-health

For a *U.S. News & World Report* article on inflammation, visit https://health.usnews.com/health-news/family-health/articles/2009/11/02/chronic-inflammation-reduce-it-to-protect-your-health.

Chapter 4

To learn more about how fluroide varnish has helped me preserve my own smile, as well as the smile of countless patients, please visit pinecrest-dds.com/book-extras. To read more on fluoride varnish and its role in tooth decay prevention, visit http://www.dimensionsofdentalhygiene.com/2015/03_march/features/fluoride%E2%80%99s_role_in_caries_prevention.aspx.

Chapter 5

To receive more information on tooth grinding solutions, visit: www.pinecrestdds.com/book-extras.

To learn more about bruxism studies and the damage from teeth grinding, visit http://jada.ada.org/article/S0002-8177(14)62575-7/abstract.

Chapter 8

For more on available sleep apnea solutions, visit www.pinecrestdds.com/book-extras.

Read the bus crash story of the sleepy driver at https://www.reuters. com/article/us-california-crash-investigation/u-s-safety-board-blames-deadly-california-bus-crash-on-two-sleepy-drivers-idUSKBNID02CB.

Learn why oral appliance therapy is often preferred to CPAP for up to 50 percent of sleep apnea sufferers: https://www.ncbi.nlm.nih.gov/pmc/articles/PMC3738032/.

Chapter 9

To see examples of dental implant succes stories, please visit pinecrest-dds.com/book-extras.

Learn about the dental implant pioneer Dr. Brånemark: https://www. nytimes.com/2014/12/28/health/per-ingvar-branemark-dental-innova-tor-dies-at-85.html.

Chapter 11

For more before and after photos of straightened smiles, visit: www. pinecrestdds.com/book-extras.

To see some case studies on how teeth straightening can improve your oral health, visit http://www.rdhmag.com/articles/print/volume-35/is-sue-6/features/oral-health-solutions-with-clear-aligner-therapy.html.

For more on braces and total health, visit www.mouthhealthy.org/en/az-topics/b/braces.

Meet Dr. Williams

Tyler Williams, D.D.S., is a full-time practicing dentist in Murray, Utah. He is a proud husband and father of three and thanks his wife, Megan, for her love and support. His kids keep him busy, and supporting his family is the driving force behind his passion for dentistry. He believes preventative and restorative dental care makes life better for families and individuals throughout the state and country. Making an impact in his community with the best health experience possible is his top priority.

Dr. Williams has studied and trained in many areas of dentistry, including prevention, dental implants, dental sleep medicine, and TMJ therapy. Dr. Williams prides himself in giving high-level care under the most ethical standards in dentistry and treating each patient as a family member. It's the experience at the office that counts. Treating teeth is important, but treating the people connected to the teeth is even more important. Dr. Williams enjoys working with his highly trained team and recognizes those who support him in his success. Dr. Williams received his bachelor's degree at the University of Utah and received his doctorate at Virginia Commonwealth University. In his spare time, he enjoys the outdoors, including cycling, mountain biking, and hiking, as well as reading. He is also an avid College Football fan.

Dr. Williams has been selected as a Top Dentist in Utah by the International Association of Dentists. He has also been awarded as one of America's Best Dentists for the past four years in a row. Dr. Williams has been featured on ABC's *Good Things Utah*, KTALK radio and in several national dental research publications, including *Dentistry Today* and the Academy of General Dentistry's *General Dentistry* journal. His practice focuses on total-health dentistry and family prevention for a better quality of life.

Contact Us:

Pinecrest Dental
463 W Murray Blvd
Murray, UT 84123

Office: (801) 618-1501
Fax: (801) 405-7709

Email: reservation@pinecrestdds.com
Web: pinecrestdds.com/book-extras

www.ingramcontent.com/pod-product-compliance
Lightning Source LLC
Chambersburg PA
CBHW071719170526
45165CB00005B/2078